Energetic Cellular Healing and Cancer

"The mind-body connection is irrefutable now, thanks to the discoveries of neuroscience. What is also uncontested is the power of personal advocacy and patient engagement in the healing process, particularly in regard to breast cancer. Tjitze de Jong takes this one step further by elucidating the link between emotions and cellular change. Pointing to how specific shifts in daily life can offset cancer's progress, Tjitze de Jong opens a portal into sustainable health care for everyone. As a neuroscientist who has specialized in resolving trauma for populations at risk, I celebrate Tjitze de Jong's book. It speaks to how individuals can act courageously to step into the center of their own health care through awareness, consciousness, and subtle adjustments in lifestyle. This brings not only hope but real physiological change through the mind-body communication networks that are innate in all of us."

— STEPHANIE MINES, Ph.D., founder of the TARA Approach for the Resolution of Shock and Trauma and author of *New Frontiers in Sensory Integration* and *They Were Families: How War Comes Home*

"Psychologist Dr. Hans Eysenck demonstrated that 75 percent of people who died of cancer had lifelong depression, 15 percent had lifelong anger, and 9 percent had both! This is just one medical confirmation of Tjitze de Jong's work. You cannot afford the luxury of anger, guilt, anxiety, or depression. The answer is energetic cellular healing!"

— C. NORMAN SHEALY, M.D., Ph.D., founding president of the American Holistic Medical Association

"Tjitze is a wonderful person, a phenomenal complementary energy healer, and now he turns out to be an engaging author on a tough topic as well. The notion that cancer may develop as a result of self-harming beliefs for as welcome news to everyone. Those who a to healing and health will be enriched by the i ts of those who have gone before in this impo g and Cancer."

— LISETTE SCHUITEMAKER, Brennan Healing Science graduate and author of *The Childhood Conclusions Fix*

"In an almost exaggerated fashion, the cancer discussion concentrates on physical problems, without taking into account the emotional, social, energetic, and even spiritual aspects which are at play. This often leads to a rather tension-filled fight against our own body, whereas these other elements of our daily existence can bring a deeper connectedness and liberate our potential toward self-healing. In *Energetic Cellular Healing and Cancer,* you can tap into a nuanced viewpoint of all aspects of illness. This book contains quite a unique combination of theory, practical examples, and exercises and opens up a path toward a holistic approach and a deeper trust in your powers of self-healing and the wisdom of your body."

— HENK FRANSEN, M.D. (Netherlands), has accompanied individuals with cancer for more than 30 years, specializing in researching and supporting his clients' self-healing potential

Energetic Cellular Healing and Cancer

TREATING THE EMOTIONAL IMBALANCES AT THE ROOT OF DISEASE

Tjitze de Jong

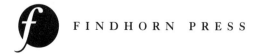

FINDHORN PRESS

Findhorn Press
One Park Street
Rochester, Vermont 05767
www.findhornpress.com

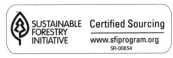

Text stock is SFI certified

Findhorn Press is a division of Inner Traditions International

Disclaimer

The information in this book is given in good faith and is neither intended to diagnose
any physical or mental condition nor to serve as a substitute for informed medical
advice or care. Please contact your health professional for medical advice and treatment.
Neither author nor publisher can be held liable by any person for any loss or damage
whatsoever which may arise from the use of this book or any of the information therein.

Cataloging-in-Publication Data for this title is available from the Library of Congress

ISBN 978-1-64411-151-2 (print)
ISBN 978-1-64411-152-9 (ebook)

Printed and bound in the United States by Lake Book Manufacturing, Inc.
The text stock is SFI certified. The Sustainable Forestry Initiative® program promotes
sustainable forest management.

10 9 8 7 6 5 4 3 2 1

Edited by Nicky Leach
Illustrations by Damian Keenan
Text design and layout by Damian Keenan
This book was typeset in Calluna, Calluna Sans, with Darwin Pro
used as a display typeface

To send correspondence to the author of this book, mail a first-class letter to the
author c/o Inner Traditions • Bear & Company, One Park Street, Rochester,
VT05767, USA, and we will forward the communication, or contact the author directly
at **www.tjitzedejong.com**

Contents

PART III: Cancer and Emotional Imbalances

PART IV: How to Heal or Prevent Illness

"Is it not the case with those who are

miraculously healed, that it is simply their expression

in the faith of miracle that heals them?"

— UMBERTO ECO, *The Mysterious Flame*
of Queen Loana

An Important
Word of Caution

The information in this book is for informational purposes only. Even if you have experience using healing techniques that incorporate the aura and chakras, if you have not studied the specific methods outlined, please do not try to apply them without first undergoing specialized training with an accredited teacher who can help you learn and practise these skills.

It is particularly important to take certain precautions when treating people with cancer. All physical cells benefit from energetic healing, and cancerous cells are no exception. Cancer spreads, or metastasizes, through multiplication of malignant cancerous cells; therefore, in order to treat somebody with cancer, it is crucial to take steps to isolate the cancerous area before running energy through the body. If you do not do this, the cancer can increase, even with the best of intentions from the healer.

It's a controversial point, which is often hard to accept in healers' circles. I've heard of and observed several detrimental examples over the years. For example, a man on his deathbed told his daughter, who for years had practised and taught the same healing modality as her dad, that he was convinced that their healing method had worsened his cancer.

Do try to remember this essential detail, whether you are the client or energetic healer. If you are the client, I suggest you ask your practitioner about their experience in treating cancer before committing to sessions. The adage "Better safe than sorry" is one I often quote to my students.

Foreword

It is not an accident that you are holding this book in your hands. Books like this one appear like a white feather at your feet or a butterfly upon your lap.

Energetic Cellular Healing and Cancer is more than just a book. It's an invitation. An invitation to what? To think differently, to see with fresh eyes, and to experience the world and its challenges in a new way.

I first met Tjitze de Jong on a visit to Findhorn, Scotland, about 15 years ago now. We were both speaking at a seven-day conference on healing and well-being with many inspiring presenters, hosted by the Findhorn Foundation. It was not a chance meeting.

Tjitze lives at Findhorn River Lodge on the River Findhorn. He swims in the river most days. His home is surrounded by barley fields. From his garden, you can take a short walk into a forest known to the locals as The Fairy Woods.

Tjitze is an outlier. He lives in the world in a different way from most of us. He doesn't have a mobile phone, a TV, or a car. He cycles everywhere. He cycled all the way from The Netherlands on his first visit to Findhorn.

Most of my meetings with Tjitze have happened spontaneously—not planned but orchestrated somehow. I feel uplifted and renewed each time I'm with Tjitze. Our conversations are always stimulating. I like the way he thinks.

I have many friends who have taken healing journeys with Tjitze, and who are profoundly grateful to Tjitze for his life-changing work. Many people go to Tjitze with serious, chronic conditions. He is often their last throw of the dice. Nothing has worked up until now, but they are still open for a breakthrough.

Tjitze and I met up recently at the Phoenix Café in Findhorn. We talked about his work.

"How do you describe what you do?" I asked him.

"I help people to not be afraid of their experience," he told me. "All healing is a release from fear."

Tjitze doesn't see cancer, or any other major condition, the way most of us do. He isn't afraid of cancer, that's for sure. "I don't see cancer as an illness," he told me. "Cancer is a catalyst—an opportunity for inner listening, to choose again, and to live a more authentic life."

Chances are—since this book is in your hands—you are facing a major challenge in your life now. We all do at some point. If so, I pray that you may find some inspiration and help here.

You needn't have met Tjitze in person to feel his healing presence in the following pages. May his storytelling and his sage wisdom be a blessing to you. May you too feel uplifted and renewed by your encounter with this book, this white feather, this butterfly.

Robert Holden,
author of *Shift Happens!* and
Finding Love Everywhere

Preface

In my book *Cancer: A Healer's Perspective*, the first publication about my work with cancer, the first paragraph of the conclusion states: "Once other writing projects . . . have been completed, I'll return to this subject and will expand it further, much further, including more case studies and a more in-depth description of physical, energetic, psychological, and spiritual influences on body, mind, and spirit, which result in the development and healing of cancer."

This promise has stayed with me for years.

I'm in a creative flow when writing fiction. Words erupt from an inner source, which feels almost relaxing. Writing about "work" is very different. I investigate material drawn from clients, previous studies, and outside sources, then combine scientific and experiential input to establish a coherent piece of writing. The goal is to have it make sense both to the general public, many of whom are directly or indirectly affected by cancer, and to fellow professionals who wish to work with cancer, using either mainstream or complementary medicine.

At times I've been tired of the self-imposed task. Time and time again, though, something has made me reread what I have written months or years earlier; something has made me restart and add a section. That "something", that source of determined inspiration, may have been ignited by a client's positive feedback or gratitude, by an article I have read, by a programme I have watched, or by meeting somebody walking a path overlapping mine.

Woven throughout the years of practising energetic cellular healing is my main inner calling. After working intensely for some 15 years with people who have (had) cancer, I've gathered a wealth of experience and insight into the causes and possible healing of the illness. Why has the work with this specific disorder become my main line of work, you may well ask? Often I ask myself the same question. Why do people with, for example, psychiatric imbalances, MS, or immune disorders rarely enter my treatment room?

The answer remains shrouded in mystery. For now, it is what it is, and if part of my life task lies in specializing in this particular disorder, so be it. The work serves a purpose for the people I work with and for their friends and family. The work serves a purpose for the development of my soul or for my spirit; otherwise, my passion would not have remained as strong as it has for well over 15 years now. The work certainly serves to enlighten the general public and bring global awareness to the phenomenon of cancer, its cause, its cure, and its prevention and is one of the driving forces behind my desire to publish this book.

The main insight I'd like to convey is that, in most cases, cancer is a psychosomatic illness. It's a simple statement, but one with far-reaching implications for how one might approach the disease. Starting from this premise, it can significantly change the role and position of the medical establishment and those of the various complementary approaches. It can encourage individuals (whether they have been directly affected by cancer or not) to take more responsibility for their own health and well-being by creating more balance in life and/or by creating and maintaining a stronger immune system. It is a statement that can shift the emphasis from cure to prevention.

Therein lies yet another kernel of wisdom I aim to get across: a change, an encouragement, a shift, and for these three nouns to enhance a manifested reality—a reality where cancer is no longer seen as a kind of unpredictable killer but a mere psychosomatic disease like almost any other; a reality where the layperson feels empowered, in charge of their life and destiny, and hence in charge of their health and well-being.

May this book encourage you to change your present-day cancer reality and support you as you adjust your perspective, allowing the unpredictable killer to give way to the empowered individual, now in charge of their quality of life and no longer at the mercy of an invisible enemy.

Tjitze de Jong
June 2020

Introduction

The causes of cancer are 90 percent psychosomatic. Or should that be 95 percent? 98 percent? 100 percent?

By psychosomatic, I mean that a person who is affected by the disorder displays a certain psychological imbalance, which can gradually (over several days, weeks, months or, most commonly, years) turn into a physical or somatic imbalance—in other words, into a disorder, illness, or disease.

For some 15 years now I've worked with people who have attracted cancer. Sometimes, the work comprises only one or two treatments; in most cases, though, the client and I engage in a lengthy process, sometimes lasting years. During this period, hundreds of clients have provided me with a stunning variety of experiences and insights into the origin and possible healing of cancer.

My training is not in medicine but in energy healing, which I undertook over six years at the Barbara Brennan School of Healing (BBSH) in Miami, Florida. Since then, I have often discovered strong common denominators in the various individuals who have entered my healing room with the presenting complaint of a cancer diagnosis. It is these discoveries that have made me ask the questions in the first paragraph as to origins of the disease.

Linked with this is the question of whether a psychosomatic disorder can be cured, or at least reduced in its significance, by undertaking psychological (emotional, mental, spiritual) inner work, which can positively affect the physical or somatic symptoms of cancer. My reply is an unequivocal yes!

Your energetic health or healing largely depends on what you are exposing yourself to during daily life. So the question is this: Are you choosing to live in an environment (physically, socially, culturally, spiritually) that serves your health and/or your immune system? And if you make compromises and choose to live in an environment that does not serve your health and/or your immune system, why do you make that choice? To be more blunt: Why would you live a life that undermines your health? What motivates you to choose a lifestyle that is to the detriment of your well-being? These are the questions I will be investigating in this book.

Alongside these questions run the opposing ones. What can you change in your daily life in order to retain your health and your immune system? What can you change in your daily life to regain your health and immune system, to heal your illness, be it cancer or another disorder? Sometimes the answer is pretty simple and straightforward; sometimes it is more complicated. But an answer can be found 90 percent of the time (or should that be 95 percent? 98 percent? 100 percent?).

One of the central themes of this book is that practically every physical disorder has its origins in a lack of energetic circulation, or an energetic block, including, based on my observations, cancer and the side effects of certain medical treatments.

We will be exploring this in greater detail in the book, but for now, let me offer an example of this central premise.

The year was 1999. I was living in a 350-year-old farmhouse in Dumfriesshire, Southern Scotland, where I had a massage clinic and was doing my second year of training at BBSH in the USA. I had learned during Year 1 to remove energetic blocks from the second (clouds) and from the fourth (mucous) level of a person's aura. The school recommended that their students not work with clients who'd been diagnosed with cancer, but I don't always do what I've been told.

A woman rang for sessions. She had cancer and was undergoing chemotherapy. After each treatment she had suffered severe side effects—nausea, dizzy spells, and numbness in her hands and feet—so her question was: Can you help me reduce these side effects?

At the healing school, we'd learned that chemotherapy produces energetic debris in the aura in the form of clouds and mucous. So there I was, a healer with the knowledge to possibly honour the woman's request but not allowed to treat her. Needless to say, I promised her that I'd do my best but couldn't guarantee a positive outcome.

During our first session, I applied the specific techniques as soon as possible after her dose of chemo. Lo and behold, the nasty side effects of medication failed to manifest, so we decided to repeat treatments every time she visited the hospital for chemo, and every time the result was no nausea, no dizzy spells, no numbness in her hands and feet. On one occasion, I was unable to treat her after chemotherapy because I was at my BBSH training in New Jersey, and all her symptoms returned. This is how simple and effective certain healing techniques can be for a person who has cancer and/or for someone who receives medical treatments.

These techniques can be taught or learned in a week. No kidding.

In 2007, I founded Tjitze's Energetic Cellular Healing School at my home on the banks of the River Findhorn, where I taught the ten-month Bodies of Light and eight-month Advanced Bodies of Light certification courses (I am taking a break from teaching and the school is currently closed). In addition, once a year, I teach the week-long Your Exquisite Body of Light course for the Findhorn Foundation. One week's study definitely doesn't teach you the finer points of working with cancer—that takes at least the full 18-month certification training I offered at TECHS—but by the end of the one-week course at Findhorn, participants have been taught how to energetically cleanse levels 1, 2, 3, and 4 of the aura, including the removal of the clouds and mucous I mentioned before.

Energetic cellular healing for cancer works; however, it doesn't mean that all my clients remain physically alive, as healing happens not just on the physical level. If a person passes on and feels more at peace during those final stages of life, that is also healing, very profound healing indeed.

This book is divided into four parts. In Part I, we explore the essence of energetic cellular healing. In Part II, I offer 15 stories of client healing, 13 of which come from my first-hand experiences with clients. Part III links these stories with the emotional imbalances at the root of cancer. Part IV offers a wealth of information and exercises pertaining to the prevention of cancer and other illnesses.

Of the 13 client stories in this book, some people have regained full health and some have passed on. Nobody can give you a guarantee for healing. Only you, in cooperation with certain medical and complementary professionals, can enhance your healing process, your well-being, and your immune system.

May what I have written be of benefit to you, whether you've actively been diagnosed with cancer yourself, one of your near and dear ones has been diagnosed, or you work in the field of cancer care.

PART I

Energetic Cellular Healing

1

Psychological Stress and Cancer

Research into, and theories about, what actually causes this "disease of diseases" is an ever-expanding field, so aiming to investigate how official sources view cancer and its causes, I did the simplest thing and carried out a search of "Cancer and its Causes" on the internet.

Google returned 128,000,000 results in 0.22 seconds. The top result was a link to Cancer Research UK (www.cancerresearch.uk.gov) followed by the National Cancer Institute (www.cancer.gov) in the USA. After checking both websites, you may notice that included in the American NCI listing is a section entitled "Psychological Stress and Cancer" but a hint in that direction is lacking in the UK summary.

During the three decades I've worked intensely with people (initially as a social worker in The Netherlands and Scotland and a massage practice that gracefully shifted into a healing clinic), psychological trauma or stress have featured strongly in what clients present in their life stories and physical complaints and will, therefore, play a major part in this book.

What does the NCI advocate in its findings and conclusions with regard to the above? Below, I quote the 2018 NCI fact sheet in full.

Psychological Stress and Cancer
According to the NCI

Key Points

- Psychological stress alone has not been found to cause cancer, but psychological stress that lasts a long time may affect a person's overall health and ability to cope with cancer.
- People who are better able to cope with stress have a better quality of life while they are being treated for cancer, but they do not necessarily live longer.

1. What is psychological stress?
    Psychological stress describes what people feel when they are under mental, physical, or emotional pressure. Although it is normal to

experience some psychological stress from time to time, people who experience high levels of psychological stress or who experience it repeatedly over a long period of time may develop health problems (mental and/or physical).

Stress can be caused both by daily responsibilities and routine events, as well as by more unusual events, such as trauma or illness in oneself or a close family member. When people feel that they are unable to manage or control changes caused by cancer or normal life activities, they are in distress. Distress has become increasingly recognized as a factor that can reduce the quality of life of cancer patients. There is even some evidence, that extreme stress is associated with poorer clinical outcomes. Clinical guidelines are available to help doctors assess levels of distress and help patients manage it.

This fact sheet provides a general introduction to the stress people may experience while coping with cancer. More details about specific psychological conditions related to stress can be found in the Related Resources and Selected References at the end of this fact sheet.

2. How does the body respond during stress?
   The body responds to physical, mental, or emotional pressure by releasing stress hormones (such as epinephrine and norepinephrine), which increase blood pressure, speed heart rate, and raise blood sugar levels. These changes help the person act with greater strength and speed to escape a perceived threat, a very useful and potentially life-saving instinctual chain of reactions. Research has shown, that people who experience intense and long-term (i.e. chronic) stress can suffer from digestive, fertility, and urinary problems and a weaker overall immune system. People who experience chronic stress are also more prone to viral infections such as the flu or common cold and to have headaches, sleep trouble, depression, and anxiety.

3. Can psychological stress cause cancer?
   Although stress can cause a number of physical health problems, the evidence that it can cause cancer is weak. Some studies have indicated a link between various psychological factors and an increased risk of developing cancer, but others have not.

   Apparent links between psychological stress and cancer could arise in several ways. For example, people under stress may develop certain behaviours, such as smoking, overeating, or drinking alcohol, which increase a person's risk for cancer. Someone who has a relative with cancer may have a higher risk for cancer because of a shared inherited risk factor, not because of the stress induced by the family member's diagnosis.

4. *How does psychological stress affect people who have cancer?*
People who have cancer may find the physical, emotional and social effects of the disease stressful. Those who attempt to manage their stress with risky behaviours such as smoking or drinking alcohol or who become more sedentary may have a poorer quality of life after cancer treatments. In contrast, people who are able to use effective coping strategies to deal with stress, such as relaxation and stress management techniques, have been shown to have lower levels of depression, anxiety, and symptoms related to the cancer and its treatment. However, there is no evidence, that successful management of psychological stress improves cancer survival.

Evidence from experimental studies does suggest that psychological stress can affect a tumour's ability to grow and spread. For example, some studies have shown that when mice bearing human tumours were kept confined or isolated from other mice—conditions that increase stress—their tumours were more likely to grow and spread (metastasize). In one set of experiments, tumours transplanted into the mammary fat pads of mice had much higher rates of spread to the lungs and lymph nodes of the mice that were chronically stressed than if the mice were not stressed. Studies in mice and in human cancer cells grown in the laboratory have found that the stress hormone norepinephrine, part of the body's fight-or-flight response system, may promote angiogenesis and metastasis.

In another study, women with triple-negative breast cancer who had been treated with neoadjuvent chemotherapy were asked about their use of beta-blockers, which are medications that interfere with certain stress hormones, before or during chemotherapy. Women who reported using beta blockers had a better chance of surviving their cancer treatments without a relapse than women who did not report beta blocker use. There was no difference in the groups, however, in terms of overall survival.

Although there is still no strong evidence, that stress directly affects cancer outcomes, some data does suggest that patients can develop a sense of helplessness or hopelessness when stress becomes overwhelming. This stress is associated with higher rates of death, although the mechanism for this outcome is unclear. It may be that people who feel helpless or hopeless do not seek treatment when they become ill, give up prematurely, or fail to adhere to potentially helpful therapy, engage in risky behaviour such as drug use, or do not maintain a healthy lifestyle, resulting in premature death.

How can people who have cancer learn to cope with psychological stress?

Emotional and social support can help patients learn to cope with psychological stress. Such support can reduce levels of depression, anxiety, and disease-and-treatment-related symptoms among patients. Approaches can include the following:

- Training in relaxation, meditation, or stress management
- Counseling or talk therapy
- Cancer education sessions
- Social support in a group setting
- Medications for depression or anxiety
- Exercise

More information about how cancer patients can cope with stress can be found on the PDQ ® summaries listed in the Related Resources section at the end of this fact sheet.

Some expert organizations recommend that all cancer patients be screened for distress early in the course of treatment. A number also recommended rescreening at critical points along the course of care. Healthcare providers can use a variety of screening tools, such as a distress scale or questionnaire, to gauge whether cancer patients need help managing their emotions or with other practical concerns. Patients who show moderate to severe distress are typically referred to appropriate resources, such as a clinical health psychologist, social worker, chaplain, or psychiatrist.

2

Bridging NCI Findings and
My Own Observations

The first sentence in the NCI's fact sheet, quoted in full at the end of Chapter 1, is of paramount importance: "Psychological stress alone has not been found to cause cancer, but psychological stress that lasts a long time may affect a person's overall health and ability to cope with cancer."

The statement instantly shuts the door on the significance of psychological stress as one of the root causes of cancer. It emphasizes psychological stress as a factor influencing a person's ability to cope with cancer once they have been diagnosed with the disease as well as its effect on people's overall health. That is how far the door has been left ajar—sufficiently open to allow a peek into the subtle and vague world of emotion and its influences on people's physical well-being, which is impossible to prove scientifically, according to general belief; sufficiently closed to keep possible psychological influences in the initial run-up to attracting cancer classed as a big unknown.

For the general public, the unknown is often classed as synonymous with frightening and scary. The vast majority of people hanker after the familiar and loathe taking risks of any kind. Due to fear of the unknown the vast majority refuse to, or see themselves unable to, think for themselves or decide for themselves. As a result, individuals often feel they are incapable of taking full responsibility for their own health and well-being. The functioning or malfunctioning of their own body is often shrouded in mystery. To the vast majority of people, unfamiliar factors play some kind of sinister role regarding health and unhealth, but as long as their physical body functions to a satisfactory degree, its functioning is taken for granted without needing to pay much attention to it.

People find it easier to leave "the paying attention to" in the hands of people who are in the know—or who at least give that impression by wearing a white coat, by having a string of letters behind their name, by occupying a certain role, and by approaching the patient from that position of authority.

Medical professionals just as easily occupy a position of authority over the patient. This is partly due to their historical position embedded in society, partly due to the public being happy to hand over self-responsibility to them, and partly due to patients being unable to think clearly during a stressful period of illness—often more so after a cancer diagnosis. Under such pressure, most people prefer to give as much responsibility as possible to the one qualified and respected person they can approach for advice, treatment, and cure.

⌒

As soon as I finish writing the last paragraph, a taxi pulls up. Tyres crunching on the gravel signal a new client arriving from the London area, staying in a local B&B for a week, and scheduled to receive five treatments. I save what I've written and walk to the door to welcome her. Her first sentence, when exiting the taxi: "Sorry, I'm a bit early." It is nigh on half an hour before our appointed time.

When she stretches out her hand in greeting, her body bends slightly at the waist in a gesture of subservience. Both her verbal and nonverbal expressions provide plenty of information: a low sense of self, not standing in her power, an attitude of not being deserving of taking up anybody's time or space. The intake at the beginning of the session confirms observations.

As the oldest daughter in her family, she had to be an example to her two younger siblings, often care for them, and take on a parental role. She was expected to provide, instead of being provided for. As a result, from a very early age, she'd been used to obeying, denying her own desires, and serving others, even when, as a girl, she wished or needed Mum or Dad to care for her.

In other words, she had had to suppress her own wishes, wants, and feelings for the benefit of others. Her own emotions were not allowed to be expressed.

Whenever emotions are not allowed to be expressed, the pathway through which they need to be uttered shuts down: throat and vocal channels. More often than not, this results in an instinctive subconscious and habitual tightening of the jaw muscles and jaw joint. Indeed, at the age of 18, my client had been diagnosed with depression and her dentist had told her to quit grinding her teeth.

Long-term suppression of emotions often leads to depression (whether diagnosed as such or not), tension in the jaw, and grinding teeth. In the long run, each of these psychosomatic symptoms can lead to headaches, migraines, thyroid imbalance, heartburn, and other digestive problems and, more long term, it can result in cancer. I will discuss this in more detail later on in the book.

Childhood conditioning prepared my client for an adult life of looking after people at her own expense by denying and not expressing her own longings. She didn't know what it felt like to allow someone to care for her; therefore, she chose a job as a carer of others: primary school teacher. She had cared for her younger siblings, why not continue the familiar pattern and change it from reversed parent/child role into a respectable job and earn a decent wage to boot?

The female body part most associated with caring, nurturing, and nourishing is the breast. Was it coincidental that she entered the treatment room with the presenting complaint of breast cancer? Is there a correlation between the decades of imbalance of nurturing and nourishment on the one hand and development of breast cancer on the other hand? From my experience I would answer here with a resounding yes! It's a sequence of events I have observed frequently over the years.

Can this be proven scientifically? Maybe . . . maybe not.

Will the medical profession acknowledge such a connection? Unlikely, as long as no scientific proof will be forthcoming.

As they say, one swallow does not a summer make. One case study or a series of observations do not justify a watertight conclusion—far from it. Nor do they justify a complete turnaround in the medical approach in treating cancer, from exclusively allopathic to one that includes psychological aspects. But does one approach necessarily exclude the other? More about this later.

To be included in any official medical list of the roots of cancer, there must be scientific proof of cause and effect, so it follows that official listings provide a limited viewpoint. Is it fair then to conclude that the medical profession works from a limited viewpoint regarding diagnosis and treatment of cancer? Perhaps. In my experience this is indeed the case, and many clients confirm my observations. Such experiences are not limited to one medical professional, one hospital, or one country, but are a global phenomenon.

Let's return now to the NCI fact sheet detailed at the end of Chapter 1. Bullet point three asks the essential question: "Can psychological stress cause cancer?"

It states: "Some studies have indicated a link between various psychological factors and an increased risk of developing cancer, but others have not."

Why does the medical world only rely on scientific studies and analysis of data and limit the healing approach solely to the outcome of gathered scientific and statistical material? When will common sense come into the equation?

In essence, we humans are natural beings, no different from insects, mammals, fish, or plants. Why have thousands of species gone extinct during earlier centuries? Why are thousands of species on the verge of extinction at present? Lack of natural balance interferes with their existence as they are unable to live in an imbalanced environment. When one or more aspects within the world of natural organisms become unbalanced that balance needs restoring.

Cancer is nothing more than our internal biological organism telling us it (and/or its natural environment) has grown out of balance. Was cancer the first message our body presented us with? Was cancer its first cry for help? Most likely not.

At the age of 18, my aforementioned client—let's call her Evelyn—had received very clear messages from her body: it was not happy with the way it was being treated, ignored, and taken for granted.

For example, her dentist had made her aware that she was grinding her teeth. Teeth are an important part of the digestive system: they serve as millstones to grind food into smaller, manageable pieces to make digestion and extraction of nutrients possible. Evelyn was most likely unaware of the fact that her jaw ligaments had developed such tightness and her jaw had started to clench during the night.

The dentist was right to sound the alarm and make Evelyn aware of her habit, and in doing so, shifted Evelyn's unawareness of her body dysfunction into her field of awareness. It is a professional's duty, whether medical or complementary, to educate patients or clients about their own body in order for the latter to decide whether to take steps to rebalance dysfunctional behaviour.

The second message Evelyn's body communicated was depression. When I asked if anything of significance had happened when she was 18, she disclosed that the family had moved away from the village she had grown up in, her only known home until that point. The youngest sibling had felt okay about the move, but Mum and the older two children, including my client, had hated Dad's idea, but in her authoritarian family his word was law.

Evelyn defied his authority by making the bold decision to leave the close-knit family unit. Despite being involved in a turbulent relationship, she moved in with her boyfriend. Although the decision was fully her own, it was a traumatic separation from the family, and she plummeted head over heels into split loyalty. She adored her father and had put him on a pedestal, but she was besotted with her boyfriend and had expected the world from him and the relationship. Can you imagine how events must have torn her heart to bits?

Evelyn's dentist had told her to stop grinding her teeth, but since it happened when she was asleep and occurred as a result of subconsciously suppressed emotion, how could she do that? She dealt with her depression by getting a prescription for valium from her GP, which removed the symptoms, so the doctor's approach was considered successful, but suppressed emotional baggage was pushed into a deeper crevice of the subconscious for it to fester; in other words, to corrode, or eat away surrounding tissues.

According to *Chambers 20th Century Dictionary*, one of the definitions of cancer is: "Loosely, any new malignant growth or tumour: properly, a carcinoma or disorderly growth of epithelial cells which invade an adjacent tissue and spread by the lymphatics and blood vessels to other parts of the body: any corroding evil."

Combining Evelyn's story with a simple dictionary's explanation of the word "cancer" provides a cause of the illness I come across time and time again: *Cancer is a festering of suppressed emotions, locked into the physical body, causing a gradual corrosion of healthy cells.*

How does the process of psychosomatic corroding and festering work in practice? My aim for the next chapters is to explain cause and effect, step by step.

3

Cells, Energy, and Health

—

Cancer is anger turned inward.
— teacher at Barbara Brennan School of Healing,
Miami, Florida, 2001

When students complete their hard-earned Bodies of Light certification after an intense, transformational journey of 10 months, they receive their diploma at a graduation ceremony. The diploma allows them to set up a practice and take out liability insurance so that they can officially practise the modality of Energetic Cellular Healing.

The name of the modality contains two elements: energetic/energy and cellular/cells. I will discuss both these components in detail in order to explain how, together, they create a set of circumstances through which health remains, through which health can become distorted, and through which health can be restored.

This last sentence only mentions the word "health" and not the words "illness" or "disease" or other synonyms. "Health" sounds and feels more positive. Positivity is a vitally important ingredient, which can help to restore any organism back to perfect health. For reasons of clarity for you, the reader, I do often use the word "disease" or "illness", although I would prefer to refrain from doing so.

In BBSH healing terminology, a negative mindset undermines the mental aspects of the human energy field—the third mental level of the aura and the third chakra (located above the navel in the solar plexus area). A positive mindset, however, strengthens them, and can help clear any weaknesses and distortions that occur as a result of an earlier inner process or conditioning of debilitating or limiting mental images and belief systems. An approach steeped in positivity is essential to restore an organism back to total health and vitality.

Every level of the aura and every chakra needs to function optimally in order to feed the body parts they're meant to energize. The third level of the aura and third chakra bring vital life force to the digestive system. Negative images or belief systems of any kind can have a direct impact on the person's digestion: heartburn and malfunctioning of the stomach, liver, pancreas, or small or large intestines, and the like. Also the body's ability to extract nutrition from food can be hampered. I will discuss this in more detail later.

In order to avoid repetitiveness, for more detailed information on the significance of chakras and the human aura, see Chapter 8.

What is a Cell?

Cells are basic building blocks of all living things, including us human beings. They provide structure for the body, take in nutrients from food, convert those nutrients into energy, and carry out specialized functions. Cells also contain the body's hereditary material and are capable of making copies of themselves.

All matter, and therefore all living things, consist of a combination of elements. An element is a pure substance, which means that it cannot be divided or changed into another substance. The smallest pure particle of an element is called an "atom". Matter composed of substances other than pure elements (including the material from which living cells are made) depend on the way these atoms are linked together in groups. Such a group is called a "molecule". In order to understand how a living organism is composed, it's vitally important to know the composition of pure elements that glue atoms together into molecules and, in the end, into a physical body.

The main ingredient of a human cell's physical composition is water (some 70 percent) besides molecules. Therefore 70 percent of our human body is hydrogen or water. When we look at the work of Masaru Emoto, a Japanese author and researcher whose work focused on the response of water crystals to energetic or emotional or atmospheric vibrations, it becomes clear how 70 percent of the chemical makeup of our cells, and therefore our physical body, responds equally strongly to different vibrations and influences. This is where chemistry meets energy, emotion, and atmosphere. This is how psychological influences affect our physical bodies. This is how emotional flow and circulation or emotional suppression affect our physical bodies.

Whereas Emoto observed the changes in water crystals due to atmospheric changes, other scientists investigated the effects of a change in emotions by observing heart rhythms. They witnessed that a strong emotional charge like anger or fear or anxiety can create extreme fluctuations in somebody's heart beat from an instant quickening to "missing a beat". Pleasant emotions like love or appreciation calm and stabilize the rhythm of the heart.

What occurs around the heart's rhythm also occurs around a cell. Various studies have shown that every change in emotional, energetic, or atmospheric vibration, as well as every thought, causes a series of physiological changes in nerve cells. Nerve cells contain tens of thousands of receptors, each specific to one protein or peptide. Each specific emotional charge releases its own surge of related peptides. Those peptides flow throughout our bodies and change the structure of each cell as a whole and make cells divide at times. If a new cell is being produced, it will have more of those specific receptors to match that specific peptide and less specific receptors of the kind that the original cells had not been exposed to.

This process confirms the commonly used statement "like attracts like". It means that if you expose yourself to negativity in thoughts, emotions, atmospheres, or energies, you will attract more of the same. Obviously, the same counts for positive vibes. Knowing that your body replaces each cell about every two months, you can recondition or reprogramme negatively charged cells into positive ones by changing your environment and train of thoughts, by surrounding yourself with positive-minded people, or, to stay with Emoto, to often use the words "love" and "gratitude", which create the most vibrant water crystals according to his research.

Our bodies consist of trillions of cells. The air we breathe consists of trillions of cells. The water we drink consists of trillions of cells. The food we eat consists of trillions of cells. The trillions of cells in our body regenerate in a continuous cycle of death and rebirth. They die off and renew themselves in order for our physical body to remain alive with all vital functions intact to

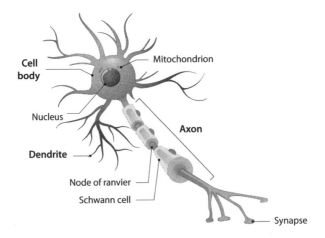

Neuron

32

survive, multiply, and keep Homo sapiens in existence. That can be seen as the original task of cell regeneration, each cell, each individual human being—the survival of the species.

In most 21st-century societies there is no apparent threat to our everyday human existence. The indirect threats of pollution, violence, rising sea levels, to name but a few, puts a knife to our throat, figuratively speaking, but the blade of the symbolic knife is not physically touching the skin. We can ignore it, organize a demonstration, sign a petition, or write to our local or national political representative. However imminent the threat may be, our daily life is relatively safe, and we're not in danger of direct annihilation. Danger no longer stems from a warring tribe, a band of raiders, or a snake hiding in the undergrowth or other directly palpable threats.

Cells die off and regenerate themselves in order for our physical body to operate optimally with all functions intact. Optimal functioning includes every nook and cranny of our body, from hair and nails to heart and nerves. In this day and age, the disturbance of the optimal scenario and surroundings is by far the biggest threat to humankind.

It's totally our own choice, especially after disturbances have been brought to our awareness (such as when the dentist informed Evelyn about her teeth grinding), whether we choose to continue disturbing our inner and outer equilibrium. Once disturbance has taken place and been brought into conscious awareness, it is also totally our own choice whether or not to undisturb the equilibrium, that is, restore our health by taking steps to rectify the body's innate, natural balance.

Health is the optimum functioning of all that we embody, including our thoughts and emotions, which allows us to live in a constant state of inner and outer equilibrium. Where inner and outer equilibrium are being disturbed, imbalance, or "un-health", can occur.

Try not to underestimate the importance of the fact that cells die off and regenerate continuously. Without it, health, even life itself, becomes impossible. Regeneration is effortless. It slips our attention totally. Do we ever think to ourselves, *It must be about time to regenerate my liver cells. Let's aim to do this over the weekend?* Surely not. We think in these terms when planning to decorate our living room or wash the car or prune bushes and hedges, but the biological organism we live in doesn't require action. Cells restore themselves in a perpetual quest for health and well-being.

Clients and students frequently ask: "If all cells of an organ, say the liver, are being replaced naturally within a week, why doesn't the liver regrow into a perfectly functioning and healthy organ? Why does it still contain imbalances as a result of, say, prolonged alcohol abuse or suppressed anger?"

Doesn't it seem a contradiction in terms, a cheat? When this is the case, why bother to eat, drink, or live healthily? What's the point of resisting enjoyable glasses of wine each evening when the habit helps us to fall asleep and forget daily struggles? What's the point of health-inducing discipline and making the effort of exercising and conscious eating and needing to go through the nuisance of sweating, showering, cooking, and washing dishes when the result remains a malfunctioning liver? Why not sit on the sofa, watch a soap on TV, whilst a takeaway pizza reheats in the microwave and the bottle has been uncorked to allow the wine to breathe?

Well, it's worth the effort! In the following section I'll try to explain this in detail, bringing together physical, emotional, mental, and spiritual aspects to paint an overall picture of a health-inducing environment that all of us can create for ourselves.

Before fulfilling my promise, let me introduce Libby, who, as a girl of seven, was not yet able to create her own environment. In my opinion, she demonstrates the epitome of psychosomatic symptoms due to emotional suppression at a very young age. It is with a heavy heart, that I recall her situation and type this.

At that stage of my career I was studying at BBSH, then still based in New Jersey in the eastern United States. I earned my income through giving massages in my clinics in Dumfriesshire, southern Scotland, and Carlisle, northern England. Libby came to see me in Carlisle.

Her mum had made the appointment, saying that her daughter had knee problems and asking whether I dealt with these things? Recalling mum's accent, it was clear that I could expect, in downgrading British terminology, a working-class mother with child. Single mother? Unemployed father? Violence? Alcoholism?

I'd witnessed plenty over the years as a social worker in a children's home in Aberdeenshire, northeastern Scotland, and during seven years as a massage therapist on both sides of the English/Scottish border. Bruises don't get massaged away—not physically, and definitely not emotionally or mentally. In preparation, I had placed two chairs opposite my own, one for mum and one for the little girl. It didn't suffice. Both parents accompanied their daughter. Never before had three people arrived for one appointment and a third chair was unavailable.

Dad claimed the comfy chair nearest the wall. He sat with his legs spread, fists planted on his hips, elbows crooked outwardly, all the while looking at me with a gaze that was defiant and demanding. His wife scurried onto the less comfortable, straight-backed chair. Her legs were tightly crossed at the ankle joints and only the tips of her toes touched the floor. Libby stood and cowered next to her, clinging onto mum's leg and standing furthest away from dad.

She was small—smaller than the average seven-year-old. Her stature was solid and stocky, more so than average. Her body appeared compressed, something I've observed frequently in Britain's working class, children and adults alike, born into a fate of obedience, back-breaking work, and at the mercy of the upper class, with no opportunity to escape. Libby exhibited a picture of centuries of oppression, gathered in one girl's body, where fear of the one in authority was obvious.

The intake revealed the girl to be riddled with allergies and skin problems, including rashes all over her body and itchy hands, but it was only her knees that bothered her. Skin problems, such as ongoing rashes and acne, indicate a wish for suppressed emotions to burst forth, beyond the skin's confines.

After the intake we explored how to possibly improve her knee. Swimming seemed plausible: movement without body weight burdening any joints. Father dismissed the option before mother was able to open her mouth: "No use. She'll sink like a brick." And when two other options were thrown out similarly, he stood up and asked how much he owed me because he had to start the five o'clock shift soon.

Baffled I protested, "But we haven't done any work yet."

"Well, get on with it," he said.

I had directed all of my intake questions in Libby's direction. She hadn't answered any. That was done for her, mainly in monosyllables. In order to draw her in, I attempted to lift her onto the couch . . . and failed. The stuckness of the working class, symbolized by her compressed body, was further accentuated by weight, a weighted-down-ness far beyond what was to be expected.

Was it any wonder I breathed a sigh of relief once the trio had left after I had massaged the extremely tight muscles in her legs? When I wrote notes on her client file, a sentence sounded out of nowhere: "She'll die of a brain tumour."

There was no reasoning behind the prediction. At that time I had not as yet treated anybody with cancer, let alone somebody with a brain tumour. I had no experience, no knowledge, no clear insight as yet into any aspect of the illness. Where, then, did this sentence surface from? From which part or parts of my subconscious? The grapevine worked well. Two years later, I heard that the spontaneous prediction had turned into truth.

⁓

Why had this sentence emerged? Without theoretical, experiential, or analytical backup, a truth far beyond knowledge had welled up in me as an inner knowing. Gradually over the years, a stronger extrasensory perception (ESP or HSP – Extra Sense Perception or High Sense Perception) has developed in me. Such sensitivity is nothing more than a method of perception we are all born with, but often fail to develop or believe in or judge it as too unspecific or too vague to take seriously.

Libby, though, from very early on in her life, had had all life force, all creatively playful force, all sense of self, crushed into a tight body. Inner breathing space was missing. Inside that girl's body, rage boiled, fed by the injustice forced upon her. Without the freedom to erupt emotionally, fury seeped through her skin. Scared of repercussions, Libby didn't dare to take a stance and kept all anger trapped inside, shielding it off in a compact armour: tight, solid, heavy. To me, this is an extreme example of energetic blocks at such a young age.

What I invite you to do is to sit still for a while, and picture Libby. Picture a girl who is inwardly as childlike and innocent and playful as any other in her age category but who is captured by fear. See if you can sense that tightness of armouring, when forced to hold all childlike impulses buried deep, deep inside. Try to notice what is happening to your emotions, your breath, your diaphragm, stomach, and pelvis. Give yourself time to let these sensations filter into your being, and witness how your body responds.

Does your breath become shallow or nigh on nonexistent? Does your head feel heavy? Do you feel compaction developing in your pelvis? Does your chest, your heart feel tighter?

See if you can spend at least 5–10 minutes in this state, and when you release it, release it fully out of your system. It is not you; it is just you experimenting. Breathe deeply, move, and feel all life force returning.

Imagine though, having to walk your life's path in a similar state. Do you really expect to escape short-term psychosomatic symptoms, such as skin or joint problems, loss of vitality? In the medium term, these can worsen into lethargy, depression, loss of libido. When such conditions are only being "cured" by symptom-suppressing medication, they keep turning inward, ever deeper, festering and corroding.

The individual remains unaware of the festering process, partly due to symptom-suppressing medication and often partly due to not wishing to know, ignoring and denying, out of fear of the unfamiliar. The bodily registration and messaging system will be functioning. The selective mind, however, will fail to register the full impact of any imbalance, not daring to acknowledge that something has mysteriously gone haywire. In the long run, a continuation of festering and corroding can turn into a full-blown disease like cancer. Most of the time, the process takes many years.

Can this be scientifically proven? Maybe . . . maybe not. If not, does such a logical sequence of developmental stages make sense? To me it does, based upon observation after observation.

4

East Meets West

After John, Paul, George and Ringo visited India during the hype and height of the Beatles' fame in the Sixties, the quartet returned to the West, influenced by the transcendental meditation techniques of Maharishi Yogi. The hippy and flower power movement followed their heroes and pioneers and picked up on it, and phenomena like meditation and yoga became cult words and initially remained activities for the long-haired, joint-smoking, and rebellious youth culture.

The youth matured, and the alternative movement shifted into widespread acceptance, incorporating all generations. Over the following decades, such activities of the subtle mind/body/spirit connection became part of the New Age movement until, nowadays, no community or activity centre offering adult education fails to include classes in meditation, yoga, tai chi, chi gong, mindfulness, and the like in their seasonal programmes.

The New Age movement emerged, basically, without much new on offer. Meditation has been practised for millennia on all five continents in different shapes and forms. Disciplines like yoga and tai chi have been a normal part of society for millennia in some eastern countries, such as India, China, and Tibet. What feels new to us in the West is old wisdom elsewhere.

Gradually, members of the public have come to include more and more beneficial elements of ancient cultures in their daily lives. As we've noticed, however, official organizations like the National Cancer Institute in the US and Cancer Research UK do not as yet include any reference to the psychological causes of cancer, let alone include the more far-reaching philosophies from different civilizations.

When institutions brush aside millennia of wisdom rooted in other cultures and class them as alternative, do they actually not take a very arrogant stance, despite the fact that many ancient techniques have proven their effectiveness for thousands of years? The two main cancer-related organizations in our Western world keep tarring all that can be learned from ancient cultures with the same brush as generations before us used to do. When they keep judging or ignoring it and remain closed to the treasures ancient wisdom can provide, they also close themselves to an open-minded and open-hearted inclusion of the connectedness between the physical body, energetic body, spirit, soul, and divinity. What does this interconnectedness actually entail? What was the root of their wisdom?

In order to illustrate the essence of interconnectedness between body-mind-spirit, I shall take Japan as an example—a country, to a large extent westernized, modernized, and industrialized, with arguably the biggest car manufacturer, Toyota, within its borders, as well as other globally renowned brand names, such as Nokia, Sony, Nissan, to name but a few. These are some of the gifts modern Japan brings to the global population. The gifts of ancient Japan can easily be covered by one single four-letter word: *hara*.

The Japanese word *hara*, which literally means "belly" but has a broader esoteric meaning, was probably introduced to the West by Karlfried Graf von Dürckheim, author of *Hara: The Vital Centre of Man*. The original title, published in 1956, was *Hara: die Erdmitte des Menschen*, which literally means "Hara: The Earth Centre of Man."

To quote Graf von Dürckheim: "By Hara, the Japanese understand an all-inclusive general attitude which enables a man to open himself to the power and wholeness of the original life force and to testify to it by the fulfilment, the meaningfulness and the mastery displayed in his own life."

In other words: "The Japanese term Hara means nothing other than the physical embodiment of the original Life centre in man."

"But, where is the centre of the body? In the region of the navel, or, to be precise, just below the navel. Therefore it should not surprise us that Hara, the essence of the vital centre, literally means belly."

"Hara is the state (*Verfassung*) in which the individual has found his primal centre, and has proven himself by it. When we speak of the state of an individual, we mean something that concerns him in his entirety, that is, something that transcends the duality of body and soul. But because man is a unity of body and soul—the body as Ludwig Klages says, being the outward form of the soul and the soul the inner import of the body—the structure of the whole individual is necessarily made apparent and legible in the form and order of his body. There is no psychic structure and inner tension that is not reflected in the body."

These quotes from Graf von Dürckheim are in essence very similar to what Barbara Brennan writes in *Hands of Light*, published over three decades later: "The individual's body is the crystallization in the physical world of the energy fields that surround and are part of each person. These energy fields contain the task of each soul. . . . The problem (task) is crystallized in the body and held there so that the individual can easily see and work with it."

Whereas Graf von Dürckheim concentrates fully on the physicalized manifestation of humankind, Brennan includes in her observations also the energetic body, aura, and chakras. The gifts she has provided to humanity through raising human consciousness via her research, writings, and teachings are invaluable. Based upon the above, you can ask yourself: "How can you experiment with such far-reaching concepts and explore how these impact your physical and subtle bodies and through that enhance your overall immune system?"

As a next step, let's explore the question that Barbara Brennan posed? You may read this as "Dare to be true to yourself". For the majority of individuals, though, it takes sheer courage to step out of line, away from society's and family's norms and values, to be true to yourself. Allow yourself to be true to yourself.

Would young Libby have dared to pluck up the courage to be herself, given her situation, still a child utterly dependent on both parents? With father ruling the roost, as he demonstrated by the way he took the most comfortable chair and sat down? Libby in her situation would have risked a clip around the ear, or worse most likely.

Of course she wouldn't dare—out of fear of abandonment as a dependent minor as well as the risk of physical, mental, and emotional repercussions. Libby would have remained obedient and not stepped out of line, trying to avoid the limelight. She would have made herself small, condensed, suppressed into an ever denser aura with chakras closed, creating an ever denser physical body. Energetically, she would have cut herself off from absorbing vital life force and would have failed to store it physically into her bodily cells. She would have reduced the function of her immune system to next to nothing and would have left herself wide open and exposed to psychosomatic symptoms. That is how Libby will have created her brain tumour and how she'll have died several years later.

Would young adult Evelyn, my earlier client, have dared to pluck up the courage to be herself? At 18, she was courageous enough to defy dad's authority, a brave step for a young adult. Bravery, though, left her at the mercy of her beloved. A way back there was not, because her father had closed the door on her, and she became financially dependent on her boyfriend as she was unable to earn her own income while studying full time. Trapped between the devil and the deep blue sea, there was no escape when it appeared that she had become the victim of a violent young man as a result of her choice to escape her authoritarian father. It was dad's suppression of her free will, which had led to Evelyn developing a teeth-grinding habit as well as depression and the risk of Valium dependency as a consequence. She had jumped from the frying pan into the fire. Her boyfriend's attitude crushed every bit of self-esteem still left in her.

Did Evelyn make a wrong choice? No. Either option would have resulted in a worsening of psychosomatic symptoms. Her choice led her body to develop breast cancer. Had she stayed at home with her father instead, she would have no doubt developed another serious illness in the long run, possibly cancer appearing in another body part.

In therapeutic circles, it is a well-known pattern people develop when they have experienced emotional, mental, physical and/or sexual abuse within their family of origin. As teenager, adolescent, or adult, they feel attracted to a partner who displays a similar domineering behaviour to the parent(s). However threatening or painful the childhood experiences may have been, they have created an energetic template in aura and chakras. A domineering partner's energetic template feels familiar, and it's precisely this sense of familiarity that results in the person feeling attracted to the prospective partner.

By daring to defy her father, Evelyn acted bravely. Prior to her move, had there been any indications signalling what awaited her when moving in with her boyfriend? Could she have registered signs of another disaster looming around the corner? Most likely there will have been. We'll never know. If there had been, would she have taken heed? Her move made it seem that she was being true to herself by following the impulse of love and making a fresh start away from underneath her father's crushing wings. How could Evelyn have known, whether she was true to herself?

Consider in this context the words of Graf von Dürckheim: "There is no psychic structure and no inner tension which is not reflected in the body."

Or consider in this context Barbara Brennan's words: "Your body holds the answer to the question: How do you know when you are true to yourself and when not?"

Taking these quotes into consideration, Evelyn's body will have held the key to a solution with less complicated and far-reaching consequences. In order to unravel a possibly smoother option, a process of listening to her body may have been beneficial. Sitting in quietude and feeling which of the two options or which other plausible alternative might have lifted her spirit could have been the answer.

Which option might have lifted her depressed state of being? Which choice could have felt lighter for a tight jaw joint? But, in the state she was in, facing a heart-wrenching decision, who in her place would have come up with such an unusual idea?

For the vast majority of people facing a predicament such as Evelyn's, sitting still and listening seems a very unlikely option. Who in their right mind would think of sitting still and listening under stressful circumstances? Also for the vast majority it would seem a very undesirable option. Stillness may bring clarity, but initially it confronts the person head on with the emotionally painful situation of the present. The emotional turmoil brings pain, confusion, and is not conducive to any sensible solution.

If Evelyn would have contemplated such a step at all, could it have made a difference? Probably not. There are not many individuals in present-day society who are familiar with inner listening or who consider themselves well versed in the skill. Why then raise this option, you may think?

Okay, I invite you to ponder the following scenarios for at least five minutes. Try and feel in your body, in your breath, in whatever physical sensations your body may convey to you, how your inner self reacts to the two options available for Evelyn.

Imagine that you stand in Evelyn's shoes on her described crossroads of life. On the left, your father and family of origin, your roots, including the often unconsciously stored loyalty of generations. On the right, your boyfriend, your love, who promises Heaven on Earth and who symbolizes liberation from suppression.

Try to spend at least five minutes visualizing each option. Your body may require more time to absorb, feel, adjust, and shift into energetic and physical responsiveness, and for your inner sensory organs to register those very responses. This is especially true when the process of inner listening is new for you. Please take your time.

Practice creates mastery. As a result of honest and diligent practice, once you master or begin to master the art of inner listening, you're internalizing an inner barometer, an extrasensory organ, registering and signalling to your own true self if and when something in you (in your body, in your emotional world, in your mental images and belief systems, in your spiritual connectedness with the divine) is amiss and out of balance.

Once you are able to register or observe an imbalance and adjust life accordingly, many a long-term discomfort may be prevented. To add a cliché: prevention is the best cure.

If, however, your physical body does present you with an illness, then the illness is only a message from your body, making you aware, that you are forgetting to be true to yourself and most likely have forgotten for quite some time. In this case, inner listening can provide a clue to the cause of the illness, and thereby a clue to its cure. Cancer is no different from other illnesses in this respect. Cancer is only a message from your body, making you aware that you're forgetting to be true to yourself and have done so for quite some time.

5

Character Defence Structures

Wilhelm Reich, a former student of Sigmund Freud and renowned practising psychiatrist, discovered by observing his patients that the specific physical shape an adult comes to embody correlates closely with the stage of childhood development during which an impactful trauma occurred. Trauma is locked into the child's body from that moment on, and over the years becomes frozen into the adult's attitude to life, their behavioural patterns, and their internalized images and belief systems. Reich called this phenomenon "Character Defence Structure".

In the 1933 publication of his ground-breaking work *Character Analysis,* Reich states: "Economically, the character in ordinary life and the character resistance in analysis serve the same function: that of avoiding unpleasure, of establishing and maintaining a psychic equilibrium—neurotic though it may be, and finally that of absorbing repressed energies."

In other words, the adult has integrated a defensive system into the physical body so as not to feel "unpleasure"—generally, fear and/or pain in their various shapes and forms. Which fears or pains people wish to avoid depends on the type of trauma they experienced and when the initial arrest of childhood development happened.

Reich classified Character Defence Structures in five categories:

* the Schizoid Defence
* the Oral Defence
* the Masochistic Defence
* the Psychopathic Defence
* the Rigid Defence

What follows is a brief description of the main characteristics of Reich's defensive quintet. For more detailed information, please refer to the References section at the end of the book.

Schizoid Defence

For the child who displays the Schizoid Defence, the "arrest", or traumatic experience, happens in the womb, during birth, or directly after birth. At this early stage in human development, the baby is focused entirely on the delicate task of entering the physical world, and if anything feels threatening, it directly implies a threat to life itself. Hence, the baby's initial impression is: Life itself is threatening.

The defensive impulse is to escape the threat; in other words, escape life itself. It does so in a subconsciously held pattern of leaving the body energetically and not grounding (rooting) into the earth—body and Earth are too physical to even contemplate.

THE RESULT: The individual has a delicate body, often displaying thin, elongated limbs and hands and fingers, feet, and toes with a tendency to feel the cold. An underdeveloped root centre (root chakra) fails to absorb physically supporting Earth energies, affecting the overall immune system of the growing child, maturing adolescent, and adult. The person may frequently suffer from joint problems, especially in legs and feet, arms and hands, or from spinal misalignments.

Oral Defence

The word "oral" says it all. The trauma occurs when the child's nurturing and/or feeding is affected. Its survival solely depends on being fed and nourished. If the supply of food is interrupted, the infant experiences it as a death threat. The defensive pattern is to grab hold of any outer source of nurturing and develop dependencies, whether that's on food, energy, attention, or time.

Basically, the person grows up relying on other people to provide for a gaping inner emptiness. Any kind of addiction can more often than not be traced to an oral trauma. The same thing accounts for eating disorders.

THE RESULT: The person displays a posture of victimhood, subconsciously targeting other people's pity: a hollow chest, shoulders slightly slumped forward, and relatively big eyes.

Masochistic Defence

For people who embody masochistic tendencies, their developmental arrest has occurred around the ages of three, four, or five years old, the time when the child develops a sense of their own individual identity, separate from father and mother. They discover their own uniqueness, for example, in creativity, and the toddler may draw wonderful pictures and build amazing structures—at least, unique, wonderful, and amazing according to its own perception.

If the child is praised and encouraged by parents, siblings, teachers, and other children, a sense of worth and uniqueness develops and creative impulses grow, together with a positive sense of self-esteem. If not, the child learns to keep a lid on creativity and their own uniqueness, because if they show their essence, criticism, ridicule, or humiliation may follow.

THE RESULT: The child learns to hide their true self, and that true self is stored, suppressed, and hidden in the seat of creativity, the pelvic region. Layer upon layer of physical protection will gradually be shaped around this area, creating a physical body that carries padding—excess weight around hips and pelvis. Mentally or emotionally, the person learns to hold in expression of the self, developing low self-esteem and is silent and withdrawn in groups. They will tend to agree with others so as not to rock the boat and avoid the spotlight being placed on them.

Psychopathic Defence

The wounding of the child who develops a psychopathic defence happens around the same age as that with masochistic tendencies, around three, four, five, or maybe slightly older. The child feels a special bond with one of the parents, senses this to be mutual, and gains a certain status as a result—at least, a status in their own mind. The child feels special and powerful as a result and will do almost anything to strengthen and confirm the status, perhaps, for example, side with that particular parent against the other parent. Gender makes no difference here, in my experience.

The position of power needs to be maintained for the child's sense of security. They will develop tactics and strategies to enhance, stabilize, or increase their power. One of these tactics is overpowering others in order to remain in control, often resulting in cheating, lying, and bullying.

THE RESULT: Over the years, the individual's body exhibits a posture of broad shoulders, a head that tips slightly forward, and hard, often penetrating eyes. The creature depicting the posture accurately is the Minotaur from Greek mythology.

Rigid Defence

For people who hold a mainly rigid defence, wounding has occurred when their heart has been deeply hurt by the first time they opened to love only to be rejected or denied. The age at which this takes place varies greatly. The emotional pain the child or teenager feels is so devastating they make a promise to themselves to never again create such vulnerability in life.

As a result, the person goes through life without emotional involvement or attachment and feels nothing, neither unpleasant nor pleasant feelings. In order to facilitate this state of being, life (surroundings, appearances, home, garden, career, car and every other aspect of daily life) is kept in rigid order: neat, tidy, and immaculate.

THE RESULT: Their body depicts balance and perfection, straightness of spine and posture.

In General

Nobody in my experience is 100 percent Schizoid, Oral, Masochistic, Psychopathic, or Rigid. Each individual has been hurt in many ways during various stages of life and therefore embodies a combination of defensive patterns.

The unravelling of the different traits and defensive tendencies is in itself a unique journey of dawning self-discovery—quite an adventure—and I can recommend to anyone to explore the self in this fashion. Your self-knowledge, and most definitely your self-acceptance and self-compassion, will increase rapidly, and you may well come several steps closer to becoming your own best friend, enhancing a sense of inner peace.

Whereas Wilhelm Reich limited his observations to the physical appearance of his patients, bodywork pioneers after him, such as Alexander Lowen, John Pierrakos, and Barbara Brennan, gradually started to incorporate the more subtle energetic body into their work. Using strong extrasensory perceptive powers, they observed how aura and chakras functioned or malfunctioned through the defensive patterns of avoiding the displeasure of fear and pain. As far as I am aware, the latest publication to delve into the five defence structures is *The Childhood Conclusions Fix* by Lisette Schuitemaker.

There have been many pioneers in the various fields of expertise of prevention and recovery from illness, but Reich, Lowen, Pierrakos, and Brennan were the four who were able to create a bridge between scientific studies and observations and subtle energy awareness in the body. As such, they were instrumental in allowing both components to merge to a lesser or greater degree in relation to prevention of illness, diagnosis of illness and recovery of health—a necessary meeting of worlds for patients' benefit.

The quartet to me illustrates beautifully the shift from generation to generation. Step by step, the old pioneering psychiatric school of Freud and Reich, with its focus primarily on psychoanalysis, began to incorporate a more holistic (whole-istic) approach—emphasis on *incorporating*, with neither of the two seemingly opposite poles excluded.

In her book *Mary Had Stretch Marks*, Miriam Connor describes the process she and her two children faced when her husband Shay was diagnosed with cancer. It is a touching story, filled with Irish down-to-earth humour. At the beginning of chapter 9, Connor writes:

> Medicine uses statistical evidence to guide treatment. The moment that Shay decided to step outside the box of expectation, he stopped qualifying as a statistic. This posed a problem with our communication with the doctors; their prediction didn't automatically apply to Shay. Research does not allow for individuals taking a different approach. We would have loved to share, to ask, to explore. Mostly we nodded and said nothing.
>
> Shay and I had no desire to reject Western medicine. We welcomed any possibility that increased Shay's chances to stay. Why does it become an issue of all or nothing, rather than the best of both approaches? It's about listening to our bodies, not anyone else.

That final sentence, with its all-encompassing significance, is vitally important. *Call No Man Master* is the title of a New Age self-help book by Joyce Collin-Smith. In my opinion, the title relates to both medical and complementary practitioners you may consult. Allow your own body to serve as your master in all possible decisions, especially decisions regarding your health. Your body knows best; your mind knows very little—unless, that is, you've mastered the art of unravelling your true self from a programmed, defended self, as discussed earlier in this chapter.

It often happens that a client with cancer receives clear scan results after a series of energetic cellular healings; however, when they try to explain to the oncologist why they think that is, the oncologist typically replies that they, as a medical doctor, have made a vow not to acknowledge treatments and their effects until they can be scientifically proven. Such a statement, however understandable and justifiable from the medical point of view, prevents any possibility of bridging the divide between conventional and complementary approaches. Does the medical professional's statement open the door to cooperation between conventional and complementary approaches? No, and that is exactly what I wish to see established during future decades.

Having said that, among the general population, an evolution in thinking regarding the use of complementary medicine has occurred in the past decade, and nowadays, my wish for alternative approaches to healing is more likely to be fulfilled. Yoga, tai chi, and meditation have earned an acknowledged place in Western society, as I wrote earlier. I have no doubt that energetic cellular healing will follow, once science is able to prove the links between disease and energetic distortions, emotional imbalances, and psychosomatic symptoms. It's only one step further in the evolutionary path of humankind and that of the health profession.

The term "Energetic Cellular Healing" refers to the branch of healing I have studied and which I practise and teach. It is the term I have given to what my work has developed into after graduation from the Barbara Brennan School of Healing. Many other terms cover related modalities of healing work, and some may well be more or similarly effective.

How does energetic cellular healing actually work? The following chapter is dedicated to answering this question.

6

Energetic Cellular Healing

In 1995, I happened upon Barbara Brennan's first published book *Hands of Light* among only five self-help books in the small Lockerbie public library in southwest Scotland, where a year earlier I had started a massage clinic. During massage treatments with clients, strange, inexplicable phenomena had started to occur and the physical massage went far beyond what I had expected. I found myself pulling black strings out of clients' throats, noticing a black cloud drifting out of a handbag and dissolving through the ceiling; a client even claimed that I had lifted a spell off her, which her grandmother (seemingly a recognized witch) had cast on her at birth. Such phenomena presented a riddle, and part of me began to doubt my own sanity. Professional credibility didn't even enter the equation at that stage. In hindsight, I can see how these years were my pioneering stage.

When I read Barbara Brennan's book, it explained matters to a certain extent, and several weeks later, out of curiosity, I flew to Denver, Colorado, to participate in an introductory weekend to her healing school. I enrolled in and graduated from BBSH in 2001, and four years later continued with the Advanced Studies programme to reach Teacher level. Directly afterwards, in 2007, I founded Tjitze's Energetic Cellular Healing School in Scotland. I felt a clear vocation with the work as soon as I sensed the possibilities of Barbara Brennan's approach: a merger of the physical with the emotional, mental, and spiritual realms. I have remained dedicated to this calling ever since.

The Essence of Energetic Cellular Healing

Two of the healer's main tasks are to hold a stronger energy frequency than the client, because energy, like water, flows from the highest to the lowest point and for any fear, doubt, or insecurity in the client to be replaced by hope and positivity.

First and foremost, it is our responsibility as healers to embody a higher frequency of energy than the client. If not, the healer drains energy away from the client, depleting their energy field instead of rejuvenating it. A depleted energy field is not conducive to healing and zaps the immune system. Practitioners have a duty to embody some state of inner equilibrium, which assures clients they will be treated with light, love, compassion, and positivity during treatments.

How do we as healers raise our energy? A multitude of tools are available, including:

- Increase our breath, both in depth and speed.
- Ground ourselves deeply in order to receive the earth's charge.
- Invoke spirit guides, (guardian) angels, or other spiritual entities.
- Set our intention to perform the healing for the highest good of the client, all of humanity, or all of creation.
- Make sure that we are in good health as well as reasonably fit, with an expanded aura and open chakras at the appointed time.

Secondly, a healer needs to remain positive in the face of a client's illness—even more so when cancer is involved, due to the strong fear element associated with the disease in our society. For many people, a cancer diagnosis is synonymous with a death sentence, preceded by a long and dreary road of suffering for patient as well as family and close friends. Additionally, they may have received a medical prediction that the illness is terminal, with a life expectancy of no more than a few months or, at best, a few years. A cancer diagnosis grips patient and social surroundings in a stranglehold of fear and/ or hopelessness.

How do we remain hopeful and positive as healers and not slide alongside the client into the depths of despair? We must know from deep within and/ or from experience that healing is always possible, even when death seems imminent.

My first ever client, Sylvia, whom I supported through a lengthy cancer journey, personified my perfect start (her story is included in full in Part II). Our work together resulted in her being fully restored to health after knocking on death's door as a result of her lower three chakras and her lower three levels of the aura starting to dissolve.

Being actively involved in her recovery has reassured me of the unlimited possibilities of healing at any stage, including in some cases, death. When a client does die of cancer after a series of sessions, many issues may have been healed and the person can pass on in peace. Sad and upsetting as this may still be for family and friends, the reassurance that healing has taken place can lighten the grieving process. A couple of examples will be mentioned later. The significance of the work of an energetic healer for people with cancer and their loved ones is not to be underestimated. To be in a position to fulfil such an intimate task for so many strangers is a tremendous privilege. Speaking for myself, these aspects of the healing work continually lift my spirit, as well as serving humanity on the physical and higher spiritual levels, and I feel deep gratitude.

How can I remain positive, even when being bombarded by fear-filled stories full of suffering day after day? Years of inner development have contributed to my present-day state of being, as well as the transformational journeys of clients I have been privileged to witness. High-frequency energies can heal whatever has been locked inside the body, clogging up unresolved issues and creating low-frequency energetic blocks.

Developments continue to extend non-medical, that is, non-invasive, possibilities in approaching both maintaining health and treating ill health. The pioneer work of Lowen, Pierrakos, Brennan, and many others taught us about the human energy field, or aura, and the perception of the body's main energy centres known by their ancient Sanskrit name of chakras, whether measured with equipment or by an individual's extrasensory perception. Pioneers lead the way for others to walk in their footsteps and move beyond their predecessors.

This is also the case with regard to cancer in both the medical world and that of energetic healing, and in the way subtle forms of energies are proven to have a direct effect on cellular activities. Examples of such subtleties are human emotions, positivity, energy frequencies, music, or a certain tone.

Let's briefly explore three very different findings based around this concept. The three researchers reach similar conclusions, although each investigation comes from a different angle.

Scientist Gregg Braden's Findings

In the YouTube video "Cancer Cured in Three Minutes", best-selling author and scientific researcher Gregg Braden, who is internationally renowned as a pioneer in bridging science, spirituality, and the human potential, analyzes what has been filmed in a medicine-free hospital in China.

A woman lies in a hospital bed with an inoperable tumour. You can see for yourself how an ultra-sound scanner is being run over her body. On a split screen, we see two images: one of the existing tumour and the other showing what is happening in real time inside the woman's body. Three practitioners stand at her bedside and chant a certain word. This word establishes the positive viewpoint in the patient that healing has already taken place; in other words, she is healthy. The trio don't see her as someone with an illness but as somebody in full health, and they convey that message to her. The patient absorbs the positive affirmation. Simultaneously, the real-life side of the screen shows the tumour shrinking and disappearing in front of everybody's eyes, including those of the patient, who is conscious throughout. The dissolving of the tumour takes just three minutes.

The implications are that the body can respond in a healing manner to positive words and phrases and energies, either from the person with the illness or others, be they professionals, friends, or family members.

Take a moment to compare this setting with the general approach in Western hospitals, where most patients with cancer are being bombarded with doom-and-gloom scenarios, with pictures of the most negative outcome possible, with fear-inducing prognoses, with the prospect of a short remaining lifespan of suffering and agony.

The YouTube video mirrors my own experiences; namely, that it is vitally important to never lose sight of the fact that any kind of cancer can be healed in a split second, regardless of how far advanced it is or how many areas of the body are affected. Once the client embraces the healing process fully all cancer can vanish, for it no longer has any reason to exist within the person's body.

Dr. Masaru Emoto's Findings

In his publication *The True Power of Water*, the late Japanese author and researcher Masaru Emoto wrote extensively about the effect of pleasant vibrations on cellular activity in comparison to the effect of unpleasant vibrations. As in the video in the Chinese hospital discussed above, he experimented with certain words, but also with different kinds of music and concluded that water absorbs information. He photographed frozen water crystals, which had been exposed to a specific word or a specific melody. The results were staggering.

The most intricately beautiful pattern emerged when water crystals had been exposed to the words Love and Gratitude. The water crystals exposed to the word Stress shrank. The water crystals exposed to the word Worrying were murkier on the edges and gave an impression of withdrawing into their shells. Water crystals exposed to Pachelbel's "Canon in D major" displayed stunningly elegant, bright, silvery shapes. Heavy metal music created a murky brownish-yellow, shapeless mass.

Water makes up over 70 percent of people's bodies. If more than 70 percent of our physical body responds to environmental influences in similar fashion to Emoto's water crystals, then it goes without saying that words coming from a positive intention and music based upon graceful beauty affect people's energies (aura and chakras), and therefore people's bodies. Everything in and around the body flows more abundantly energetically and physically.

Not only water and people, though—also milk and cows, apparently. Several decades ago, I cycled through Luxembourg and took shelter in a shed when a rather heavy shower tried to dampen my mood. Well over 100 dairy cows wandered around freely inside, and there was not a person in sight. To my surprise, music flowed from several speakers. The farmer's intention was clear. Through the relaxing influence of J.S. Bach's Brandenburg Concertos, he intended to improve the mood in the dairy herd and increase the flow of milk.

Gregg Braden and Dr. Masaru Emoto's findings are linked by the phenomenon of increased flow of energies, or in other words, higher frequencies of energies. The healing words of the three men in the Chinese hospital had largely the same effect as the positive environment created by Emoto. The spontaneous disappearance of the tumour and the pictured water crystals have been exposed to higher frequencies of energy and respond accordingly. This leads to my third example.

Bruce Tainio's Findings

While working for Eastern Washington University in Cheny, Washington, in the United States, the late microbiologist Bruce Tainio, founder of Tainio Technology, built the first frequency monitor and began to measure people's frequencies in different states of being. He recorded the following:

* Healthy body frequency: 62–72 Hz.
* Genius brain frequency: 80–82 Hz.
* Normal brain frequency: 72 Hz.
* Colds and flu start at: 57–60 Hz.
* Disease starts at: 58 Hz.
* Candida overgrowth starts at: 55 Hz.
* Receptivity to Epstein Barr disease starts at: 52 Hz.
* Receptivity to cancer starts at: 42 Hz.
* Death starts at: 25 Hz.

When I first read about these measurements, I was fascinated. My immediate thought was: *If I live at a more or less continuous high level of energetic frequency, the chance of illness reduces significantly.* My second thought was: *If the average person lives more often than not within a high-frequency field, the chance of remaining healthy increases.*

And then a third thought, linking all three findings: *If illness depicts or needs a low frequency to begin its development or continue its existence (cancer starts at 42 Hz.), health can return by inducing high frequencies of energy into or onto the patient. The three Chinese practitioners give us a clear and very direct example of how high frequencies resolve a tumour.*

7

DNA and the Future
of Energy Medicine

The abbreviation DNA stands for Deoxyribonucleic Acid. Such a concoction of letters is gobbledygook to me, as it may be to most readers. Still, we come across these three letters practically on a daily basis.

In a nutshell, DNA is the hereditary material in humans and almost all other organisms. Nearly every cell in a person's body contains the same DNA, the information for all that we humans embody, feel, think, and connect with, which is stored as a code made up of four chemical bases. These bases pair up with each other and create a strand (a ladder-like, elongated spiral structure) unique for each individual.

Gradually, humanity is coming to grips with the fact that DNA may well hold the key to our genetic makeup. Does it also hold the key to our health, unhealth, and healing?

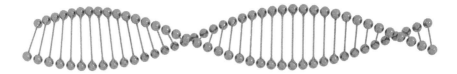

DNA strand

It has been proven recently that emotions affect DNA strands. For a more specific explanation, I invite you to read Barbie Zabel's blog "Science Says DNA Can Be Changed with Feelings" (https://barbiezabel.blogspot.com/search?q=science+says+DNA). For more information on experiments regarding emotions and DNA, check out the work of Dr. Vladimir Poponin (www.researchgate.net), the US military, and the Institute of Heart Math (www.heartmath.org).

Dr. Vladimir Poponin believes that his discoveries have tremendous significance for the explanation and deeper understanding of the mechanics underlying subtle energy phenomena, including many of the observed alternative healing modalities. One of the revolutionary experiments is called "DNA Phantom Effect". It concludes that (a) a type of energy exists that has previously gone unrecognized, and (b) cells and DNA influence matter through this form of energy.

Using controlled laboratory conditions, Poponin and his team of researchers found that changes in DNA changed the behaviour of light particles—the essence of our entire world with all that exists in it. Their work shows the powerful relationship between specific frequencies of energy and specific states of well-being, something that ancient traditions have known for centuries.

Scientific discoveries like these show ancient healing methods in a very different light and validate their potential. As millennia-old wisdom from the East meets Western science, the chasm between both worlds narrows and sturdier bridges between them are built.

Studies have shown that when a healing practitioner's energetic field is in harmony, as described earlier, their aura and chakras expand and DNA strands shift positively. This influences the energy flow and frequency of the physical body. Automatically, the healer's presence raises the frequency of the client's aura and chakras, as well as the energy frequency of their physical body, in a process called "harmonic induction", which describes the effect of one field/tone/frequency on another. This is not unlike the action of a tuning fork, which with its sensitivity to vibration makes this phenomenon easily visible. Why would such sensitivity limit itself to a mere metal structure? Well, it doesn't. Each aura of each object or living being shows the same capacity to tune the frequency of another, just as a tuning fork does.

One of the essences of energetic healing is that the subtle phenomenon of harmonic induction works to improve health by positively affecting DNA.

It is the bridge that links Gregg Braden's theories of healing, as exemplified by the filmed three-minute cancer cure in the Chinese cancer hospital, with the water molecule experiments of Dr. Masuro Emoto and the energy frequency measurements of Dr. Bruce Tainio.

Simply put, for an ill person—who has a low energy frequency—to be in the company of a person embodying a significantly higher frequency is already a healing experience. This is why participants and students wish to remain close to a teacher or guru during meditation, yoga, or tai chi classes. The energy field of a person practising such disciplines regularly has been measured to be of a considerably higher frequency than that of a layperson. For this reason, it is one of the main responsibilities of practitioners of energetic healing to embody a higher frequency of energy than their client.

The three exciting scientific discoveries I noted above have important implications for the future of energy medicine as they can be linked to recent insights about the sensitivity of DNA strands. Do these discoveries hold the key to our health and well-being? If so, we may be able to make a revolutionary shift away from pharmaceutical approaches to healing illnesses and diseases, be they cancer or any other malady, as well as preventing them from taking hold in the first place.

In the Sixties, the Beatles were instrumental in introducing Eastern approaches to well-being into mainstream Western society. Now, half a century later, we've moved onwards and upwards. Science is gradually building and strengthening a bridge between Eastern and Western concepts of health and unhealth, and the apex of that bridge, which is still under construction, is energy and energetic transmission.

Another pioneering experiment during the same Sixties decade acknowledged the vital importance of energetic vibrations and transmissions. The spiritual community of Findhorn in Scotland was started organically by Eileen Caddy and her husband Peter and their friend Dorothy Maclean and grew way beyond expectation. When unexpectedly made redundant they started growing vegetables to subsidize their diet. Their focus at the beginning was on successful gardening in poor soil conditions, using spiritual guidance received by Eileen Caddy and Dorothy Maclean from the elemental forces of devas and the angelic realm. The three founders discovered through experimenting how energetic frequencies were of paramount importance for the growth of vegetables, herbs, flowers and even composting. As described in the 1976 book *The Findhorn Garden: Pioneering a New Vision of Humanity and Nature in Cooperation*, Eileen's spirit guides during the beginning stages of creating the gardens suggested:

> It is necessary to work with the soil, to love the soil and feel it alive in your hands. When it is not alive, bring it to life with love and tenderness, with care and feeling. All of this brings you closer to the things that really matter in life.

And this was her very human reaction to the guidance:

> We were told that each of us had a particular kind of radiation to give to the soil and the garden. Quite honestly, I hadn't a clue what "radiations" were. It didn't mean a thing to me, but this is what

kept on coming in guidance. We were told that it was frightfully important—"Not only for now in what you are doing for this garden, but it is for the reconstruction of this earth"—so I would go out into the garden to work, trying to keep in mind that I was putting radiations into the soil and plants. Then one day when I was spreading compost, I became totally concentrated on what I was doing and I could actually feel the life force flowing through me. I knew that I was doing more than helping the plants and soil just physically.

The transformation Eileen went through during this process is as simple as it is stunning. From a woman who was utterly unfamiliar with gardening and energetic radiation, she showed unwavering faith in her spiritual connection and guides. She followed their guidance to the letter and served as a human bridge between the esoteric, spiritual realms and the physical world of gardening.

The Findhorn experiment brings us back full circle to the practice of Energetic Cellular Healing and to the practitioner and his responsibilities. Following on from the revolutionary theories and experiments in the previous paragraphs, we'll explore specific elements of healing skills in order to complete the picture of this particular form of energy healing.

8

Healing Techniques

This chapter contains a fair amount of theory and aims to describe the nature and working of the various healing techniques I apply on a daily basis. In Part II, I will tell client stories in more detail and frequently refer to these different healing modalities. At that point, seeing the techniques placed in a real-life context, the following explanations will make more sense.

Our energy body contains seven major *chakras* (energy centres or "wheels of light" as is the literal meaning of the Sanskrit word) and an *aura* (human energy field) comprising seven corresponding layers, or levels. Ideally, chakras rotate clockwise to absorb energy from the surrounding area (the universal energy field), feeding the various auric layers and the physical body. The bright and expanded aura functions like a buffer zone, filtering out illness-inducing energies, so that the body absorbs only health-enhancing energies, thereby helping the body to maintain its healthy equilibrium.

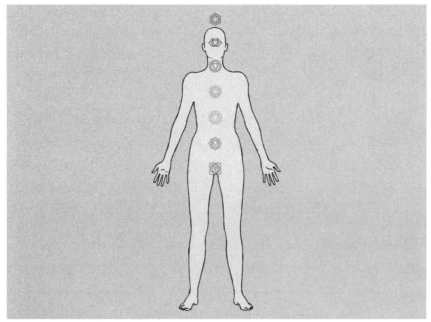

Chakra System

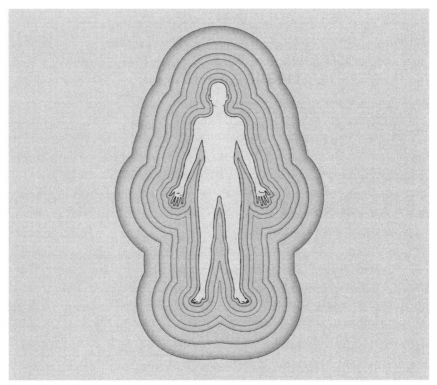

Aura or Energy Body

Unfortunately, ideal circumstances rarely exist in modern society, especially not long term. As a result, one or more chakras may be dysfunctional. Ideally symmetrically cone-shaped, a chakra may be misshapen, spinning counter clockwise, or not spinning at all, preventing the aura from maintaining its clean, clear, and expanded state. As a result, the physical body is prevented from absorbing the necessary energy frequencies in order to maintain full and vibrant health. Any distortion in the physical body (illness or its onset) is preceded by an energetic imbalance of chakras and aura. Prevention of illness means keeping aura and chakras in balance as well as keeping the physical body in good shape. Healing the root cause of illness requires restoring aura and chakras (body, emotion, mind, spirit) to their innate balanced state, as well as treating symptoms in the physical body.

HSP or ESP

Before I try to describe and explain some of the healing techniques I apply during sessions, let's first explain another main healing tool: HSP (High Sense Perception) or ESP (Extrasensory Perception). Both abbreviations and terms cover the same phenomenon. Our familiar five sensory organs (eyes, ears, nose, skin, tongue) are definitely not the only gateways with which to perceive our environment. Alongside the physical sensations of seeing, hearing, smelling, feeling and tasting, we also have access to the same five senses non-physically, through extrasensory perception.

Each individual has this capacity. Children tap into it more easily, but the more they are taught and conditioned to develop their analytical capabilities, the further ESP is being pushed into the background until it's no longer accessible for most people. Artists, clairvoyants, shamans, and the like have never lost their childhood capacity, or they have relearned how to tap into these sources of information.

In my case, I had to relearn it.

Prior to finding Barbara Brennan's book *Hands of Light*, in which she describes HSP in great detail, I had started a massage clinic. Treatments consisted solely of physical touch, and as far as I was aware, in my ignorance at the time, there was no exchange of energy. That concept never even crossed my mind. HSP developed spontaneously, and due to my unfamiliarity with energetic healing, I had no idea what was happening, what I was tapping into, or what was being released and healed spontaneously.

As I noted earlier, when I worked with one woman who found it a challenge to speak her truth it felt as if I was pulling black strings out of her throat. Did I remove part of the energetic block that made verbal expression difficult for her?

Then a male client asked if I'd be willing to treat his wife, who seemed to attract every virus or infection out there due to a weakened immune system since childhood. After our first and second sessions she felt somewhat better. Then, during the third treatment, whilst I was working on her neck, out of the corner of my eyes I watched as what looked like a black cloud lifted out of her handbag, hovered upward, and slowly disappeared through the ceiling. Cold shivers ran down my spine, but I quietly kept massaging.

Afterwards, I asked whether she had noticed anything special when I'd worked on her neck. She had, but chose to first discuss matters with her husband. I was very curious on her return the following week. Her explanation: "My grandmother, who was a recognized witch, put a spell on me when I was born. That's why I always felt poorly. You've removed that spell and I'm okay now." She paid, left, and we never met again.

On a third occasion, I worked with a young mother who felt grief over aborting her first pregnancy. When she sat opposite me, crying, much to my amazement a non-embodied human shape appeared adjacent to her chair. It looked like a boy, about six or seven years of age. When I asked whether the abortion had taken place that many years ago, she looked up in surprise and confirmed my HSP. It was as if I saw streamers of energy flowing between mother and son. I reported this back to her, and she sensed a strong, loving light appearing in the room. The occurrence supported and eased her grieving process immensely.

These three unusual events left me puzzled. I noticed that clients benefited far beyond what could be expected from massage, but I had no explanation at that time—it would come after I enrolled at the Barbara Brennan School of Healing for my four years of study. During that time, my HSP developed just enough to graduate each year of my training, but because I had to fit into the highly structured framework of the educational organization, with all the criteria I had to fulfil in order to achieve a certain standard, spontaneity ebbed, and my personality missed that. It was only when I began teaching several years after graduation, and found myself supervising whole groups and classes, that my HSP began to grow stronger. HSP or ESP is not some kind of mystical power that only a few privileged people use. High Sense Perception is a kind of sensitivity you too have been born with and can develop.

What follows is a short summary of some of the techniques involved in Energetic Cellular Healing, whether aimed at cancer treatment or the treatment of any other spiritual, mental, emotional, or physical imbalance or any combination thereof:

* Restructuring chakras
* Restructuring organs
* Clearing and charging relational cords
* Cleansing and strengthening auric levels
* Spiritual surgery

Restructuring Chakras

As noted earlier, a chakra is a cone-shaped "wheel of light" absorbing vital life force, or energy, from our surroundings by spinning in a clockwise direction. Through developing their visual HSP, a practitioner of Energetic Cellular Healing can start to notice whether there are distortions in a client's chakras.

For example, a chakra may be thin and wobbly and not securely tipped into the Vertical Power Current (VPC), or energetic line, where the seven major chakras align, or sometimes not connected with the VPC at all. A chakra can also be reduced in diameter or not reaching out into the world in a straight line; instead, it may be hanging downwards, pointing upwards, or veering to either left or right. The chakra movement can have shifted from clockwise to counter-clockwise, or it can display a horizontal, vertical, diagonal, or ellipse-shaped movement.

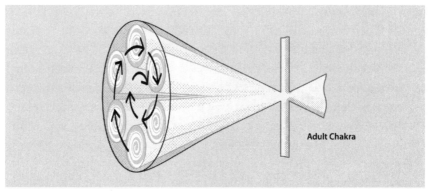

Adult Chakra

Chakra cone

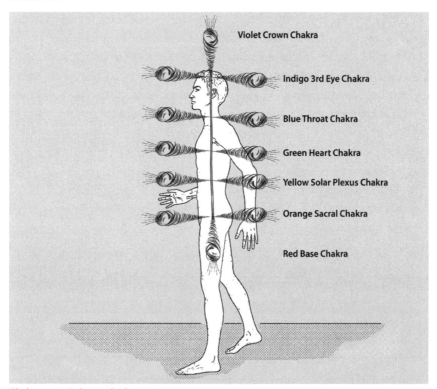

Violet Crown Chakra

Indigo 3rd Eye Chakra

Blue Throat Chakra

Green Heart Chakra

Yellow Solar Plexus Chakra

Orange Sacral Chakra

Red Base Chakra

Chakra cones in human body

All of these distortions have a physical, emotional mental, and/or spiritual significance, and their misalignment causes a reduction or distorted energy absorption that must be repaired if the energy body is to supply our body with health-enhancing vitality. In my experience, this is one of the most effective healing techniques I perform.

For people with cancer, however far removed or close to death they may be in their disease process, it is vitally important to strengthen the immune system, because cancer is often synonymous with a death sentence in people's mindset. For example, the first chakra (the root chakra) energizes the overall immune system, so restructuring the root can give a real boost to the person's physical energy and to their outlook on life. Embedded in the root chakra is the cord that relates to the earth, the incarnational cord. When a person has no hope of recovery, this earth cord can become thin, depleted of energy, and lacking in deep-rootedness and the diseased body is unable to absorb vital earth energies necessary to remain physically as well as energetically connected to our planet; in other words, they lack the capacity and motivation to remain physically incarnated or alive.

Restructuring Organs

Every organ in the human body is surrounded and permeated by an aura comprising seven different levels, each one vibrating with a specific frequency of energy. Every level of the human aura can be cleansed, repaired, and charged, and the same is true for every auric level of an organ.

When an organ has been affected directly by cancer of the liver, the pancreas, or the kidneys, for example, I see the organ encapsulated in a dark, sometimes totally black field, which can also be visible inside part of the organ or inside the whole organ, depending on the spread of the disorder.

When the cancer is of a different nature, there's still always a noticeable impact on certain organs, especially liver and kidneys. Their function is to purify the human body by filtering blood and other fluids. Cancerous cells are toxic, and equally toxic is dead cancerous cell material. The excretion of this cancerous cellular toxicity and the alien, artificial ingredients of medication puts pressure on the human purification system. HSP indicates clearly, virtually without exception, that the organs involved function in a sluggish manner and have become overly burdened, exhausted, and require extra support.

The relief to the organ, both inside and out, is easily visible once it receives healing attention—brightness replaces dullness, and the overall energetic circulation increases. Once the liver and kidneys are functioning again, toxic cellular material may be excreted at a great rate, leading for a short while to diarrhoea, dark and smelly urine, increased perspiration, skin breaking out in spots, and the like. Uncomfortable as these short-term symptoms may be, whenever they occur for a client, I enthusiastically explain the reason: healing is happening to a degree.

Repairing Relational Cords

Within each chakra are energetic streamers connecting one individual to another. These are called relational cords. As soon as we have any kind of interaction with somebody, we develop cords between corresponding chakras in our bodies. When the two people only interact with each other in loving kindness, cords are healthy and vibrant, with positive energies flowing unhindered in both directions, and they look shiny and bright. Needless to say, this is not always the case.

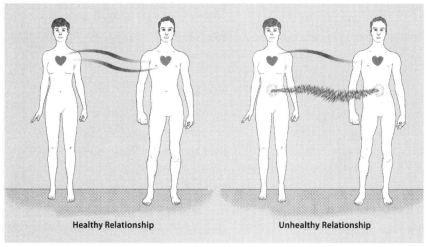

Healthy Relationship   Unhealthy Relationship

Relational cords between two people

More troubled cords can look darker, surrounded by a thin veneer of stagnated energy of a murky brown, red, yellow, or green colour, depending on the unresolved emotional issue. The energy might also flow in one direction only when one person clings onto a previous partner or wants something unspoken from the other. A cord may also reach out into empty space and be frayed at the tip indicating that somebody is unable to satisfy a certain wish or desire.

Similarly, a cord can reach out, but then curve back into the same chakra in a loop, in the case of a person living a certain repetitive life pattern, such as continuously choosing an abusive, overpowering partner. In the case of an abusive relationship, such as after sexual abuse, a cord can be connected in the second (pubic/sacral) chakra and tip into the VPC amidst a deeply embedded dark mass of stagnated energy, which can leave the person in question unable to achieve a satisfactory sexual relationship, or be unable to achieve orgasm or any other kind of sexual pleasure. Such a long-term block may lead to disease of sexual or reproductive organs, including cancer.

All of the above is visible with HSP, and cords can be cleansed of each of these distortions.

Cleansing and Strengthening Auric Levels

As noted earlier, the human aura consists of seven separate layers, or levels, corresponding with the seven main chakras. Each level has a different structure and a slightly different energetic frequency. Some levels are structured in such a way as to contain lines of light of a certain colour, along which energy pulsates continuously. These lines can be torn, thin, frayed, or the spaces in between the lines can be too wide (absorbing negative energies too easily) or too narrow or dense (not allowing for the absorption of positive energies).

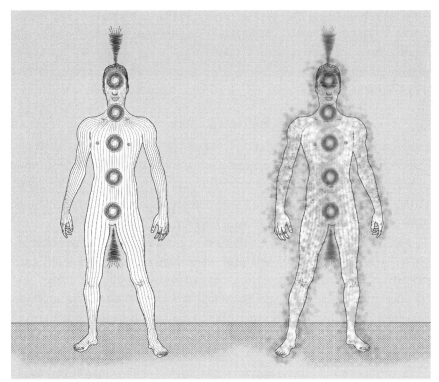

Structured level (left) and unstructured level (right) of the aura

When, for example, the first chakra is weak, the lines of light on the first auric level show a similar weak pattern. When somebody's mindset is veering towards a negative outlook, the yellow lines of light in the third auric level, the mental level, are thin with little energy flowing through.

Some levels are open, unstructured spaces containing beautiful pastel colours. Distortions through emotional blocks or stagnations due to the suppression of emotions can be seen or sensed as clouds in the second auric level, the emotional level.

In this way, each level of the aura has its own structure, its own significance, its own specific imbalances, and its own method by which to repair those imbalances. The healing techniques involved are not so very complicated.

Whenever a client with cancer comes for sessions, I first do an intake with them to establish what is going on. The information I gain as a result, besides the information gained through HSP, gives me a clear indication of what the client may need, first and foremost. If chemotherapy and/or radiotherapy are involved, for instance, the aura will look dirty, murky, and dense and become more dysfunctional. That's why a medical treatment like chemotherapy can have such devastating side effects: nausea, hair loss, numbness, and lack of power in the far extremities of fingers or hands, toes, or feet. The cleansing of the various auric levels can often prevent the onset of side effects, and can therefore keep the client's quality of life intact and give them a more positive outlook on the disease process.

Spiritual Surgery

For people with a more analytical and scientific background, spiritual surgery may well be the most challenging healing technique to accept. Spiritual surgery happens when one or more non-incarnate beings, or guides, work through the healer into the client's body and perform spiritual surgery as if the person is lying on an operation table in hospital.

Most of the time, my guides let me know; I hear a voice or feel a prompting nudge or intuitively sense their urge when they wish to work. All that is required of me at that moment is to first sit down. I prefer to sit because it takes less effort to keep my hands immobile and I never know in advance how long the spiritual surgery will take. Then I place both hands on the client's body and raise my frequency by extra grounding and by an increased rate and depth of breath. Both my guides and I need to be on the same energetic frequency in order to merge and cooperate. They lower their frequency somewhat, and I increase mine until we connect. As soon as the connection has been established, my guides take over and I surrender, let go, and allow them to perform their tasks with their all-encompassing knowledge and wisdom far beyond my own insight.

Basically, the operation occurs on the fifth level, which is a template level for both lines of light of the first level and the body to fit into seamlessly. In the beginning, it totally baffled me what I witnessed: guides gently lifted the body part or the organ energetically out of the body so that it floated above the client onto the fifth level. This is where my guides operate on the client and make the necessary adjustments before ever so gently placing the energetic body part or organ back into the client's physical body. The organ literally appears to float in front of my eyes.

Clients with a certain level of sensitivity can perceive the guides' activities. One woman who had fibroids in her womb reported that she felt the guides entering her body and her womb, taking hold of the growth, cutting it away, and finally removing it.

What I see occasionally is that surgical instruments are moving through my hands and fingers or, more often, that metallic bluish ultra-thin laser beams extend from my fingers and cut into cancerous tumours. Spiritual surgery requires that levels 1–4 of the aura have been prepared thoroughly beforehand.

In General

These are the five main healing methods I utilize when using Energetic Cellular Healing to treat clients with cancer. Less frequently, I may use other techniques, such as removing minute viral or bacterial or other potentially infectious cellular material, straightening and strengthening a client's *hara* (energetic core) alignment, and unshrouding and expanding a client's core essence, or spirit's core.

As stated earlier, each of the healing techniques mentioned above can be explained, taught, and learned. It does not take "a person with special abilities" to perform such modalities; only somebody who passionately feels drawn to working in depth in the field of energetic healing. If you are interested in undertaking training in Energetic Cellular Healing, a list of educational institutions offering this work may be found under References.

An Important Word of Caution

I want to reiterate that the information in this book is for informational purposes only. Even if you have experience using healing techniques that incorporate the aura and chakras, if you have not studied the specific methods outlined, please do not try to apply them without first undergoing specialized training with an accredited teacher who can help you learn and practise these skills.

It is particularly important to take certain precautions when treating people with cancer. All physical cells benefit from energetic healing, and cancerous cells are no exception. Cancer spreads, or metastasizes, through multiplication of malignant cancerous cells; therefore, in order to treat somebody with cancer, it is crucial to take steps to isolate the cancerous area before running energy through the body. If you do not do this, the cancer can increase, even with the best of intentions from the healer.

It's a controversial point, which is often hard to accept in healers' circles. I've heard of and observed several detrimental examples over the years. For example, a man on his deathbed told his daughter, who for years had practised and taught the same healing modality as her dad, that he was convinced that their healing method had worsened his cancer.

Do try to remember this essential detail, whether you are the client or energetic healer. If you are the client, I suggest you ask your practitioner about their experience in treating cancer before committing to sessions. The adage "Better safe than sorry" is one I often quote to my students.

The next section of this book contains 13 client stories, information on their individual backgrounds, diagnoses, medical interventions, and some of the journey we travelled together.

PART II

Client Stories

9

Adam's Story

Type of cancer at our first session: lung cancer
Dominant character defence: rigid

The year is 2014. Next week is Easter. This means that Adam was diagnosed with cancer in both lungs exactly three years ago. We were introduced to each other by his daughter, a medical doctor who lives overseas, who had taken part in the Conscious Medicine Easter conference at the Findhorn Foundation organized by the late Gill Edwards, after the latter published her final work with the same title.

(Note: Gill's own cancer story would also have been a telling one to relate in this book, and my guess is that she would have wholeheartedly agreed to have her journey included here. However, because she was such a well-known personality, I have decided to respect her and her family's privacy by excluding her story. Bless you, dear Gill, in deep gratitude for your decades of ground-breaking work in the field of psychology and personal development and for bringing conventional and complementary medicine one step closer together. Your efforts will not be in vain—promise.)

Back to Adam. He was about 70 years old at the time we worked together, and had been a chain smoker practically all his life. He preferred convenience food over a healthy diet and television over exercise. He lived alone in a big bungalow about 50 kilometres away and barely socialized. His wife had passed away some seven years earlier.

When a person is not fully acknowledging the grief of losing a loved one and holds back its expression, the emotion is stored in the lungs, according to Louise Hay's *You Can Heal Your Life*. From my own client observations, I agree with her.

Adam was a classic example of suppressed grief. During our first couple of sessions, I made several attempts to support him in entering a grieving process to help release the dark cloud of stagnated energy that held his heart, lungs, and chest in a vice-like grip. My HSP also showed that the Vertical Power Current (see Chapter 8) had lost its central position and veered toward the back. This meant that Adam (consciously or subconsciously) avoided the front aspects of the chakras, the emotional centres. In practical terms, it meant that my client avoided emotions of any kind, a familiar pattern for somebody with a predominantly rigid character defence.

It soon became clear that the father was not as broadminded as his daughter. He aimed to escape any direct question by falling silent, staring into space, and without exception, some evasive remark followed after about 10 seconds. Explaining theory made no difference, nor did asking him to make direct eye contact with his wife through his mind's eye to support emotions surfacing, and nor did any other approach—until he made clear in an unexpected and admirable spell of clarity and assertiveness of mind that he wanted me to quit questioning him about the loss of his wife. Adam made sure to keep avoiding his feelings; what he wanted was for me to fix his cancer.

All I can do at such a moment is respect the client's wishes and explain the pros and cons of his choice. For myself, I have to make up my mind whether I deem further treatments useful or a waste of time, money, and energy. In Adam's case, after obtaining his permission first, I also consulted his daughter, and together, we decided it was beneficial for sessions to continue, with the aim of controlling the possible spread of cancer as much as possible. This decision was a key factor in Adam not having to undergo any medical treatment other than having a six-monthly scan in order to keep an eye on any internal developments.

The scene was set. Here we have a client who expects somebody else to fix the problem, and cooperation was minimal from the outset. The situation improved for short spells only after his daughter's or my encouragement, but on the whole Adam stayed passive, cycled the occasional few minutes on the home trainer, kept the grief for his late wife locked inside his lungs, only rarely went fly fishing (his main hobby in the past), hardly ever met up with friends, and turned into the classic couch potato in front of the telly in a living room stagnant with cigarette smoke.

After this summary, you might expect Adam's health and fitness to have gone downhill rapidly. And there you would be wrong. After three years, it still hasn't.

The man has grown visibly older, no doubt. What mainly holds Adam back in life is not cancer, but both hips, especially the right hip joint, which suffers from a considerable amount of wear and tear. It makes him unstable and insecure on his feet and prone to slip and fall. Instability can be a risk factor when fishing on a riverbank, where grass and rocks are often slippery underfoot and the current can be strong and dangerous, especially when the river is running high.

Why then does the cancer not progress to a level that makes life miserable for a man who consciously chooses each day to not set a strong intention to improve his own life's quality?

Whilst it's true that he consistently ignores advice and prompting from both his daughter and me, carries on smoking and living a sedentary life, and undergoes no medical procedures of any kind, here's the thing: his life is not ruled by cancer.

From other stories you'll read here—and likely those you'll hear from your relatives, friends, and media—you may have gained the impression that the journey through cancer is a particularly tough one, ruled by suffering, fear, hospital appointments, anxious waiting times for scan results, insecurities regarding health and life itself, or seemingly imminent death approaching. Yet Adam has refused any medical intervention. Is this a deciding factor in maintaining a stable quality of life? Sure, his hair is thinning and he is losing strength in both legs, but then again, both symptoms are to be expected of a man his age.

If he were to enter the medical arena, he'd encounter doctors, radiologists, oncologists, specialists, and consultants and would likely ricochet from one to the other. Health and life are thus at the mercy of a team of people in authority. It takes a person with strong assertiveness to stand his ground during daunting consultations, when the dreaded prognosis and diagnosis is being delivered. Most of the time, to protect themselves and the system they represent, the medical consultant is prone to paint a worst-case scenario in order to cover all eventualities. Statistical data and percentages can come across as a threat and may give a patient the impression that they've been reduced to an impersonal number on a conveyor belt. The minds of most patients may run riot with all the "what ifs", even if the survival percentage they receive seems pretty high. The maelstrom of thoughts is almost always either fear-inducing or fear-enhancing.

Adam made a conscious choice, influenced by his daughter, to not undergo active medical treatments. Despite the fact that he is doing very little to enhance his own health, the cancer has barely progressed for the last three years, and the illness has practically no influence on his daily life.

His situation is not unique, but it is exceptional, considering that few people dare to make a similar decision. In that way, it has been and still is a privilege to support Adam and to keep following his progress for over three years now.

10

Archie's Story

Type of cancer at our first session: an aggressive form of sarcoma,
with cancer in the left buttock, spine, ribs, and both lungs
Dominant character defence: masochistic

Occasionally, I share a story of my work with a cancer client on Facebook, obviously making sure confidentiality is being respected. It is because of one of these posts that one of Archie's family members recommended the man get in touch with me.

When he contacted me, as luck would have it, I had a space in my diary the very next week due to a cancellation. He and his wife acted speedily, made travel arrangements, booked a bed-and-breakfast, and I met them just several days after our initial telephone conversation.

It turned out that our first meeting was just a fortnight after he had received his cancer diagnosis, and quite a diagnosis it appeared to be. He was in his mid-thirties and had married a loving and strong wife. Their mutual respect and dedicated love stood out when I first met them. They had two children, one aged three and the other not yet six months old. It was clear that this family of four had a lot to live for. It was equally clear that both parents shared a positive outlook regarding the situation they faced, despite the medical profession giving Archie no chance of survival.

Four months earlier, Archie had begun to experience pain in his left hip and thigh, and his sleep had deteriorated as a result. As you might expect, fatigue had crept in and his immune resistance had gone downhill, which can have a negative effect on the overall immune system.

After pain in his right arm and fingers set in, his GP organized an MRI scan. The diagnosis, as noted, was a shock: Archie was found to have the most aggressive form of sarcoma, with cancer detected in his left buttock, the entire spine, ribs, and both lungs.

Most people facing such an ordeal would have hung their heads in despair and given up hope almost instantly. Not Archie and his wife. It doesn't happen often that a first meeting with a client leaves a lasting impression. The whole family had travelled up north for the visit, and the love and care exuding from all four of them was a joy to behold.

As is often the case when a new client with cancer arrives for a first treatment, the intake is a lengthy one. Questions, answers, discussions, and explorations can easily take close to an hour. The conversation creates an instant connection between healer and client, but more than that, it aims to clarify the underlying, psychosomatic cause of cancer. In addition, it provides new insights for the client on the probable why, what, and how of the disorder. The intake, therefore, may well give the client an incentive to change certain attitudes, habits, or patterns, once the penny has dropped as to why the cancer may have developed. From my perspective, the intake indicates which directions will be the most effective and beneficial for this particular client in this particular situation so that I can adjust my approach and techniques to the individual's needs.

Archie's intake was no different. He and his wife had already taken the initiative and begun exploring the issues on their own and felt that Archie's overemphasis on work was one of the reasons his life had become unbalanced. At the young age of 18, his parents had found him a flat, given him a month's rent, told him to quit his education, get a job, and look after his younger brother, who was allowed to attend university. Without too much of a grumble, Archie took his parents' orders as gospel and set to work, shouldered the responsibilities of a substitute father for his brother, threw himself into a career, and soon earned well and started to live an excessive lifestyle. Such an attitude and choices are typical of somebody with a predominantly masochistic character defence: looking after others, conforming to the norm, and fitting in with what others expect from him at the expense of his own comfort, ease, and life quality.

He did what was expected of him. Complying with other people's demands and overriding his own desires gradually caught up with him, though. Marriage and starting a young family failed to compensate, and depression kicked in, giving him little lust for life.

Another turning point came when Archie's father fell ill about 18 months prior to his son's cancer diagnosis. Again, Archie accommodated his dad's requests (or demands) and acted like his father expected him to. This time around, the demands required that Archie drop many of his daily commitments and be at his father's bedside as long and as often as the senior man felt necessary.

Whilst he complied with these parental demands, I wonder: Did Archie experience resentment, or did he wholeheartedly devote his time and energy to his father and put his own priorities on the back burner? Did resentment gnaw away deep inside, swallowed and repressed due to the son's sense of duty towards his father? As a result, did resentment fester and drain energy and possibly, unbeknownst to the young man himself, reduce his life force even further? Did this process settle the already apparent sense of depression even deeper, as deep as the bone's marrow? Did all of the above affect his immune system negatively?

Such questions can never be fully answered with a clear yes or no, as you'll find in other examples in this book. Why then include these questions and possible theories, you may wonder?

The correlation between life events and an individual's conditioned patterns on the one hand and the onset of a (serious) illness on the other remains tenuous. Even so, I invite you, the reader, to consider all possibilities with regard to cause and effect of illness. An open mind can lead to an inner journey of exploration, one in which the individual tries to unravel for himself how the apparent imbalance started and how it can be remedied.

When a client and I undertake such an exploration, I always encourage them to remain open to all possible answers or solutions, including the seemingly most far-fetched and unlikely ones. Even though my client had already embarked on an exploratory journey with his wife, we delved deeper during the intake. Explaining the why, what, and how of masochistic tendencies and their long-standing impact on health allowed more pennies to drop for Archie.

Taking into consideration the seriousness of the diagnosis, as well as the lifeline Archie had provided himself—his positive attitude supported by his marriage—I chose to apply some general healing techniques that first week: restructuring the first chakra (root chakra) and fifth level surgery, or spiritual surgery, and placing my emphasis on supporting and strengthening the client's positive energies. I was able to work on higher frequencies of energy with somebody like Archie than is possible with the average client, and he felt the high voltage vibrating through his entire body and revelled in it.

He was also alarmed by the intensity of my breath and movements at times, despite me telling him not to worry when high frequencies passed through my body, and out of care and worry for me, he placed a hand on my shoulder to make sure I was alright. Tricky though it is for me to speak during an expanded state of being, I managed to mumble that I was perfectly okay, and it underscored for me his masochistic pattern of putting other people's well-being before his own.

The six sessions that week were successful, insofar as Archie felt much better, lighter, less in pain, and freed up to a certain extent. His wife noticed and was thrilled, excited, and inspired. On their return south, she instantly enrolled for the Your Exquisite Body of Light course, the week-long workshop I facilitate annually for the Findhorn Foundation, which was due to take place four weeks later.

She almost didn't make it, though. Three weeks after our sixth session, she sent me an e-mail requesting my support. Archie was in a really bad state, and he might not survive, after having been given either an overdose of chemotherapy or the wrong type of chemo in hospital. Her husband made it through the crisis, and she was able to take part in the workshop, leaving her husband in her parents' care.

About a fortnight later, the family was due to travel north again for the next series of treatments. Having observed how Archie's wife had taken to my type of work so easily during the workshop, her husband's predicament, and how well also he responded to high-frequency work, my mind orchestrated an experiment using as inspiration the YouTube video about a healing session in a medicine-free Chinese cancer hospital (see Chapter 4 for a full report on the experiment).

To recap: the video is a perfect example of how applying a consistently positive mindset (in energetic terms, the third chakra and the third level of the aura) can dramatically improve health and well-being. A woman lies in a hospital bed. She has an 8-centimetre tumour in her bladder. Her abdomen is being monitored by a camera. A screen above the bed shows two pictures adjacent to each other. One side shows the actual tumour; the other side shows real-time events as they unfold during the session.

Three practitioners stand around her bed. The trio has been specifically trained to create the exact vibration in their hearts that corresponds to full recovery for the patient. Their vibration radiates outwards, affecting the energy field of the patient. The patient is fully conscious and believes in the unfolding process and its positive impact. Elsewhere in this book I describe the phenomenon of "harmonic induction". What I relate here is exactly that put into practice.

During the experiment, the three people repeat the one-word healing message they have agreed upon, which creates the sensation of healing and ultimate health. Basically, the three practitioners are communicating with the patient's energetic field that healing has already taken place. The woman's energy field responds effortlessly through the aforementioned harmonic induction, and the woman herself doesn't need to do a thing to instigate healing. On one half of the screen, the camera registers that the tumour shrinks and fades away altogether within three minutes.

Our impromptu treatment faced several disadvantages compared with the Chinese situation:

- Archie didn't have one tumour; he had cancerous growths in several areas.
- The three people around the bed hadn't been specifically trained.
- We didn't have the technical equipment at our disposal to monitor what was going on inside the client's body.

Prior to Archie's session, the six people gathered briefly discussed proceedings and the scene was set. Archie lay down, the three people went and sat about two metres from the treatment couch, the cameraman was prepared, and I took my seat directly adjacent to the client.

Initially, the trio repeated their healing phrases in silence. Its effect seemed barely palpable. At one point, whilst performing the usual healing techniques, I requested that the three make their voices heard, and the energy shifted remarkably.

Surges of additional healing vibes rushed through my entire system. The client's body shuddered, spasmed, and convulsed like never before. The room was filled with potency, exceeding all expectation, and the healing session turned into an awe-inspiring spectacle for all to witness and sense—so much so that after about a quarter of an hour, the cameraman, a therapist himself, put his camera down, went down on his knees, and sat in prayer. At the conclusion of the treatment, we were all left in stunned silence.

The burning question was obviously, had the client healed? Archie looked considerably lighter, younger, and unburdened, with bright shining eyes. He reported that he had experienced dark masses and energies leaving his body, confirming my sense of what had taken place. All of this is not unusual after a treatment.

Our final session for the week was scheduled for the next day. The change in Archie's cancerous areas had been significant, to say the least. I remember mentioning to him at the beginning of the healing, "There's not much for me to do today." It was quite a statement, and a sign that our experiment had been very successful—not that all cancer had been removed, but with the disadvantages we faced compared with our Chinese example, that would almost have been too much to expect.

Six weeks later, we met again for several sessions. During the interim period, Archie had obviously been back home in the London area, with all the dynamics and environmental impacts that city life brings, which is so different from life in and around Findhorn.

In his case, it also brought with it the tendency to fall back into an earlier, energy-depleting trap, namely to look after other people first (as he had once had to look after his younger brother) ignoring his own well-being. Falling back into such a familiar trap can easily stimulate the continuation of illness, not just of cancer. The familiarity of a life pattern effortlessly fits in with a physical body and an energetic body remaining in a diseased state or returning to a diseased state. Preventing the return to familiarity is recommended, therefore, if not essential during a healing process.

However, in normal daily life, that is not always an easy task, surrounded by pressures from family and friends and colleagues. What is required to heal fully at such a stage is a kind of social quarantine, whereby the client is solely surrounded by like-minded, supportive people who understand on all levels where the person in question is at and what they need for healing to fully settle into their belief system. Such an all-encompassing healing environment is not easily found.

This is where we're at at the moment of typing. The journey continues for Archie and his young family. What they've experienced is the existence of options and possibilities for healing, whereas the medical profession classes his situation as terminal. In their unique way, both husband and wife keep doing their inner therapeutic and energetic homework. They've learnt to sense and work with their chakras, auras, emotional past and programming, mindset, and so forth. In that way, I definitely see hope for the family to remain together, as do they themselves.

11

Luciana's Story

Type of cancer at our first session: third diagnosis of cancer,
initially in right breast and ribs
Dominant character defence: psychopathic combined with rigid
striving for perfection

During the first 37 years of her life, Luciana's cancer had been diagnosed three times. When she initially rang me, all of the tumours had been removed and she was receiving ongoing conventional treatments, medications, and checkups. That situation was destined to continue for the foreseeable future.

Her symptoms at that stage included blurred vision and unstable sugar levels. Her blood count was lower than expected, and each morning she awoke with a stiff left hand. Her aim was to regain full health—nothing more, nothing less.

From an early age, Luciana had had an inexplicable fear of falling victim to a serious illness and dying young, and she perceived that it was this belief that was preventing her from returning to full health. Indeed, after three encounters with cancer, she was finding that her limiting beliefs had only gained momentum and now had a stranglehold over her thought patterns.

The disease process had started three years earlier, with cancer in the right breast and two of the posterior ribs. Treatments, including mastectomy and surgical removal of lymph nodes, had been successful up to a point, but cancer had returned twice. The final operation had been six months before our first contact. Luciana described herself as a perfectionist, blessed with enormous willpower, which had supported her battle in the face of a barrage of onslaughts, a roller coaster ride of ups and downs spanning six years. Whereas many people finding themselves in that exhausting predicament for such a long time might well have waved the white flag and surrendered, Luciana's zest for life didn't allow her to give up.

The main traits of a person with a predominantly psychopathic defence are enormous willpower that allows them to easily override emotions. Competitiveness is a fact of life for them; therefore, surrendering is a rarity. Luciana displayed the characteristics of a typical psychopathic personality that relies on hypervigilance to check on everybody and everything in order to stay safe. With this in mind, especially after cancer had already returned twice, this young woman monitored every move, every breath, every intake of food and drink. Relaxation was not high on the agenda.

We began by addressing emotional issues and underlying mental concepts, images, and belief systems. For example, she believed that because she'd been able to heal her cancer at an earlier stage what she had done should yield positive results for others. Thus, when a neighbour attracted cancer and point blank refused to follow Luciana's advice, she had felt very frustrated. She had the common sense not to bombard the neighbour openly with her beliefs, knowing from experience how that might affect the person in question, and instead, had suppressed her frustration, stored it energetically as well as physically, and offloaded it verbally in my presence.

For me, this was a striking example of how the direction one chooses to take in maintaining health and treating illness is a purely individual matter. Luciana's advice had been given with the best of intentions at heart, but what she at that instant (like most people) failed to take into consideration was that each individual travels an individual journey and takes responsibility for the decisions throughout life according to their own priorities and beliefs.

We may be aware of this rationally, but when it is played out in real life amongst our circle of acquaintances, friends, or family, we lose sight of it when we feel the emotional charge of painful helplessness. When that helplessness is accentuated by our friend's refusal to accept the shred of help on offer, we may well feel frustrated. My suggestion is that if you encounter such an attitude, bring to mind the Serenity Prayer, used by Twelve Step programmes like Alcoholics Anonymous all over the world, and this may reduce any feelings of frustration:

> God, grant me the serenity to accept the things I cannot change,
> the courage to change the things I can, and the wisdom to know the
> difference.

To put it differently: everyone's reason for becoming ill is different, and so is the path they need to take in order to return to health and vitality. That path is nobody else's. Different people can take the same path for a while, but at a certain turnoff or crossroads, the individual paths diverge as a result of different decisions they make. The parting of paths may be forever or for a short distance only.

My client Luciana, for example, walked a different path from her neighbour. Her life purpose was different. Their only common ground was that they were both human beings with an illness called cancer who lived in the same geographical area. Their reasons for becoming ill were different, so their decisions about which path to take to regain health differed.

I have no idea what decisions her neighbour made regarding her cancer treatment, but Luciana's decisions indicated a broad approach of combining conventional treatment of medication, operations, and scans with a complementary approach that included acupuncture, bioenergetic healing, nutrition, massage, and shiatsu and support from her local Maggie's Centre, where she could drop in whenever she needed information and support on her cancer journey.

Some people may judge her approach as over the top. Some may prefer to keep decisions in the hands of those who are traditionally expected to know about such things—the medical profession. And some may question who or what contributed most to my client healing her cancer twice before and form their view based on this.

Luciana's view is simple: if something feels right it's beneficial, and if the practitioner feels right they will be of benefit to her. Does it matter which elements of the overall package contributed more or less to her health? Not in Luciana's view. She asked questions, felt an absolute right to do so, and ultimately, each practitioner she chose was of benefit to her health. The questions she asked allowed her to choose the people she wanted to have around her during her cancer journey, find the right fit for her health team, her crew, and she herself remained at the helm, steering her vessel according to her compass readings, according to her path. She was both skipper and leader, highly energized and motivated, just as you might expect from a true psychopathic character.

Our first series of sessions focused on cleansing energetic and physical bodies, with the aim of minimizing the chances of her cancer returning. In hospital, blood tests were carried out every six weeks to check her malignant cell count. Her initial score was 4.4, and at 5.0, she remained within the risk zone.

In lay terms, the blood count I am referring to is a tool to evaluate the various sorts of cells in the blood. The number and size and distribution of these cells can give lots of information about a person's health status, including bone marrow function; nutrition and alcohol status; hydration state; blood loss; medication effect; liver, spleen, and kidney function; infection; inflammation; and cancers.

With her cell count thus close to the danger area, Luciana never felt she could relax her strict regime, including diet. She was strong-willed, as noted earlier, which pressurized her into rigid discipline. Fun things like going out for meals and anything that might disturb the daily balance of activity and rest were kept in check, but as a result of this rigid attitude, partly necessary and partly self-imposed, pleasure was missing as was the balance between duty and relaxation.

In other words, Luciana barely allowed herself to live; instead, she was being lived. Life was dominated by treatments, be they conventional or complementary; by tests and the stress of waiting for results, whether positive or negative; by dietary restrictions; by the need to sleep and rest much more than this sporty woman wished; by visits to Maggie's Centre; and by so much else.

After working together for several sessions, it was clear to me that Luciana was fed up with having cancer and needing to consider the possibility that it might return. She was utterly fed up with having had cancer for so many years and not being allowed to lead a normal life to prevent its return.

Looking back at her file, I can see that our eighth session together was a turning point. My notes say:

Strong light from the start and L. surrendering deeply. Very, very intricate
5th level work. (I'm referring to spiritual surgery, see Chapter 8)
  1. Blood on higher frequency, stronger immune system.
  2. Guides taking bad cells out of frog-spawn-like mass, creating more space
     for light in chest cavity. and L.'s breath responding each time.
     L. very tired afterwards and may enter healing crisis. Possible detox.

Several treatments and three months of gradual improvements followed. There is so much to gain on so many levels if and when a predominantly psychopathic person starts a process of waving the white flag and surrendering. Luciana began to radiate more health, well-being, and light. A consultation with her oncologist undermined the progress temporarily and instilled fear in her. He expressed caution regarding the scan results. His cautiousness undermined Luciana's already fragile sense of trust, made fear flare up, and afterwards her aura had visibly contracted.

Kidneys store fear. They are located directly below the adrenal glands, which, amongst other hormones, produce adrenaline, a hormone essential for our instinctive flight-or-fight response during times of danger. Following her visit with her oncologist, the aura of Luciana's kidneys had responded by clouding and contracting energetically and Luciana's physical body had followed the fluctuations inside her aura, with the result that her kidneys' ability to filter toxins from her blood cells had been compromised.

This is an entirely natural phenomenon. Imagine a flower bud or leaf in springtime. When temperatures and sap rise, the aura of the plant extends and creates an energetic mould for the flower or leaf to grow into. Take a moment to sense or see this happening. It can be a fun and educational way to develop or check your visual HSP.

The next time I saw Luciana, she had just returned from a holiday in Greece, and the warmth and sunshine and our session signalled another period of renewed hope, energy, and increased vitality for her. Within a week, she had received the message from three independent sources that all traces of cancer had vanished: a medical intuitive, a healer colleague, and me.

Around the same time, her sister gave birth. I do not recall whether it was her sister's first baby and my client had become an auntie for the first time; significant, though, was that Luciana's desire to become a mother reignited—pregnancy, childbirth, breastfeeding, and motherhood. She had removed all thoughts of having a child from her mind after three episodes of breast cancer and the removal of one of her breasts, but true to her inquisitive nature, she searched the internet and discovered that her wish was not as outlandish as it seemed. Many mothers have given birth and breast-fed babies after healing their cancer, including those who have undergone a mastectomy. Not surprisingly, as soon as she set this intention, more energy gathered in her womb and ovaries, as if her body was giving her the thumbs up.

After a couple of months of inner contemplation and talking over the idea with her husband and me, she took the bull by the horns and discussed her wish to become a mother with her oncologist. He was baffled. His expectation was that Luciana would take medication for the rest of her life and he doubted whether her periods or fertility could or would return.

Needless to say, his patient was of a different opinion. Dependency on anybody or anything was not her style, and definitely not dependency on any kind of medication. This was even more true now, because medication was preventing Luciana's periods from returning, making it impossible for her to become pregnant. After further discussions and some time had passed, the oncologist opened up to the idea and proposed a plan with regard to her medication regime.

During this time, Luciana wondered whether to sign up for my 10-month Bodies of Light training. This training is an intense journey, a deeply delving, transformational therapeutic process that teaches students intricate healing techniques related to our physical and energetic bodies. Over the years, about 50 percent of participants start a private healing practice or use the training to enhance another modality; the other half join for self-development. The class can be a tremendous boost for the immune system and self-awareness, bringing together wisdom, knowledge, and experience in order to learn how to strengthen, cleanse, and repair their own aura and chakras.

Luciana would not have been the first person with a history of cancer to participate; however, allowing a person with a history of cancer to take the course can be risky. Energy healing stimulates cellular activity and can therefore also stimulate activity of cancerous cells, which needs to be prevented at all cost, and students do work on each other in class, practising various techniques. For that reason, as recommended by one of the teachers during the fourth and final year of study at BBSH and mentioned earlier, it is essential to energetically isolate the cancerous area to avoid multiplication of malignant cells. It's a simple yet sensitive skill. The healer needs well-developed ESP in order to be able to check and make sure that isolation has been achieved prior to running energy through the client's body. Beginning students cannot be expected to display such a high degree of sensitivity.

I will allow some clients whose cancer has been removed and healed, by whatever means, to sign up for the Bodies of Light programme, but not others. The person's safety is the deciding factor. When the client feels like they have integrated the healing process on all levels (physical, emotional, mental, spiritual), then participation can only be health-enhancing. If this is not the case, I will decline their request and explain why I am postponing their participation on the course. Ruthless honesty is important. If the decision is unclear to me, I err on the side of "Better safe than sorry". I need to feel a resounding and indisputable yes within in my heart and soul; if I do not, something is amiss somehow. I cannot afford to put the client at risk, and to a lesser degree, my professional reputation.

In Luciana's case, when I listened to my inner voice, I heard an unreserved yes with regard to her taking the course, so between August 2009 and May 2010, our relationship changed from client/healer to student/teacher. (Note: In order not to confuse roles, I do not give individual treatments to Bodies of Light students.) I scrupulously supervised her progress throughout the course, and no complications occurred. She achieved all of the necessary skills to pass her certification training and graduated with a well-earned diploma.

During the first two years after graduation, I saw Luciana for six sessions. In a nutshell, her risk factors went down, MRI scans remained clear, hormonal medication was stopped, her periods returned, and more energy gathered in and around her reproductive organs. The oncologist was ecstatic that one of his patients had become a walking miracle.

These positive factors didn't make Luciana sit back and relax, though. That wasn't her style. Besides that, she felt frustrated inwardly—frustrated by the slow recovery and the ever-present risk of the illness rearing its head for a fourth time, exacerbated by her inexplicable life-long fear of dying young and the need to remain vigilant. She was frustrated mainly by not being able to work and contribute to society and her joint marital income; the latter increased after her husband was made redundant.

All of the above contributed to a continuous level of resistance, frustration, and general pissed-off-ness in my client with what life threw at her. Rarely was I able to welcome a truly happy, light-hearted, or trouble-free woman when she arrived for a treatment, despite her being "a walking miracle". That wasn't enough for her. Sometimes I wondered whether any achievement would suffice, or would her innate drive to reach more or higher goals keep pressurizing, if not pestering, her?

Was this ever-present inner turmoil the psychological explanation behind the fact that 17 months after graduating from the Bodies of Light programme, a scan showed up tiny fragments of activated cancer cells in various body parts, mainly the lungs and vertebrae? Because they were minute and not gathered in one place, the medical profession was unable to tackle them. Luciana was devastated. All fears had been confirmed.

My diary did not open up to see Luciana until two weeks later, when we scheduled four sessions in one week. This is not unusual. To make the cost of travelling (time, energy, and expenses) worthwhile for clients from further afield, we often book a series of sessions close together. For example, at the time of writing, a client from Germany has received five healings this week; next week, a woman from England has four sessions booked, and in a fortnight's time, a Swedish woman has reserved eight slots.

Fear and devastation bombarded Luciana. She rarely relaxed, and mental tension showed strongly in the third and mental level of her aura. In a mentally relaxed, active person the level consists of bright yellow lines of light, pulsating with energy and extending somewhere between 8 and 20 centimetres from the skin. The level reflects beliefs, ideas, thought forms, and perceptions.

During the fortnight before I was able to see Luciana, the lines of light had received a hammering from her mind running overtime and focusing on fear, insecurity, and negative concepts. Scary scenarios that had chased her from childhood onwards had morphed into harsh reality for a fourth time, and the effects were obvious. A healthy pulsation was absent, and the lines had turned brittle and thin and unable to conduct much energy. In turn, mental chaos filters down into the lower auric levels and affects the second and first layer of the aura, directly adjacent to the skin. This ultimately prevents health-inducing energies from being absorbed by the physical body. Distortions with similar consequences can appear in each of the seven auric layers. Each auric layer indicates an imbalance of a different aspect in a person's life.

The four treatments were successful in helping Luciana to feel lighter, less scared, and more hopeful and positive, and both client and I felt that the cancer had been significantly reduced. My guides confirmed my perception during the last session. It was also apparent that not all unease and disease had been tackled.

After those sessions, I did not see Luciana for four months, due to my busy teaching schedule of workshops and Bodies of Light trainings and a month-long work trip in Hong Kong. When we were finally back in contact, by phone initially, an avalanche of bad tidings ensued, and when we met, Luciana had lost a considerable amount of weight due to lack of appetite and to cancer eating away at her insides.

During my absence, cancer had been diagnosed in both of her lungs, spine, brain, both hip bones, and particles had been traced floating in the blood. The area around the right lung and the heart showed fluid retention, and Luciana kept coughing. Her hips ached, and she felt constantly tired and drowsy. The walking miracle had dropped back to Earth with a big bang, a devastatingly big bang steeped in harsh reality. Needless to say, her entire being was flooded with a strong existential fear. More than anything, it was the diagnosis of cancer in the brain, which rattled any positivity out of the woman.

One negative aspect of being strong-willed was that Luciana had not slowed down or allowed herself to relax once cancer had retreated for a third time. One benefit of being strong-willed, though, was that, even under these severe circumstances, somewhere deep inside, Luciana found the willpower to not let the illness get the better of her. Of all my clients in the 20 years I've had my own clinic, if there is one person who deserves a gold medal for fighting spirit, it's Luciana. I have often admiringly wondered how she kept going, especially after receiving such an incredible blow for a fourth time.

So, she searched on the internet and found a German cancer clinic. Their methods claimed to gain very positive results. She wanted to go there at all costs. Friends chipped in with donations to make the trip financially possible. She was deemed too weak to travel initially, but once she had regained a bit of strength, she went several months later.

In the meantime, the NHS prescribed chemotherapy and Herceptin. Luciana simply hated having to go back on medication, undergoing all the horrible tests and scans again, and the far-reaching implications of cancer returning. It was everything that had previously filled her with frustration about the inability to lead an easygoing, full, and fulfilling life. Why had she been living such a restricted life? What had been its use if all roads ultimately lead back to cancer? What had been the point? What was the point of life, anyway, when it all ended in disease, fear, and agony, with all of it only postponing death itself, as a foregone conclusion, its arrival postponed by an agonizingly long road of suffering? Luciana simply hated that motherhood would now certainly pass her by. The ultimate feminine creative force was not hers to experience. She had a lot to come to terms with.

This spirited woman consulted a specialist in London who designed a healing programme for her. She consulted a medical intuitive and herbalist in a town near me. She asked friends who were travelling to the world-renowned healer John of God in Brazil to take a photograph of her to show him, and request distant healing. She received and took many supplements and returned to a strict diet.

Did Luciana clutch at straws? It never felt like it. Despite her fear level being very high, she took steps to think things through and consider alternatives and always made enquiries before making a final decision as to whether to consult a particular practitioner.

We brainstormed alternatives when we met. We worked on dissipating fear as much as possible. We worked on regaining hope and positivity, when sometimes there seemed no reason to have any. We worked on stimulating her immune system by restructuring her root chakra time and time again. We worked on balancing and strengthening the other chakras. We worked on cleansing and energizing the seven levels of the aura, partly to reduce any unpleasant side effects of chemo. We worked with both of our spirit guides and raised energy frequencies often to allow them to perform spiritual surgery.

Cooperation was made easier by Luciana having completed the Bodies of Light training. She understood what we were doing, and my language and actions made sense to this intelligent and aware woman. We formed a strong team, supported by a deep level of mutual trust and respect, and each fortnight a double session was scheduled.

Within six months, scans indicated that the cancer was retreating. Her lungs only contained tiny specks of active cancer. Her brain was cancer-free, which meant, that Luciana's biggest source of fear was letting go of its stranglehold over her. Her bones, spine, and especially her hips healed more slowly, which was to be expected, since the skeleton is the densest part of human anatomy and thus, the most stubborn to shift shape.

For a while the skin of both of her hands yellowed, a clear sign that the liver was working overtime to cope with the alien substances the body had to deal with: medication, supplements, chemo, blood transfusions, and cancerous cells dying off. The liver is the body's most powerful cleansing agent, and it needed support, so we spent a fair amount of time restructuring the organ in our sessions.

More than a year after the devastating fourth diagnosis, Luciana dreamed that all was clear. A biofeedback machine also indicated that all was clear, and my sense was similar. Guides told me that there no longer was any need to isolate cancerous body parts, because the high risk of cancer spreading had vanished, despite minuscule traces of cancer still being detected in her lungs and hip bones.

This more or less brings us up to date with Luciana's present situation. She is well. Her body is practically cancer-free again. She has returned to her reputation of being a walking miracle. Her oncologist is once again ecstatic. The last scare had a strong impact on Luciana after years of a healthy existence and graduation from Bodies of Light, so I don't expect that she will ever fully relax. The ghost of cancer returning will take a lot of taming before she will allow herself to believe that it has been laid to rest forever. Each time a scan is due, she is nervous. Each time results are due, she is scared. But she lives and has energy and can lead a pretty normal life.

I've debated whether to write this final paragraph because when I recall the fragment of conversation Luciana and I had about six months ago, the lump returns to my throat and tears burn in my eye sockets. Luciana pursued so many different approaches after the fourth cancer diagnosis that I found it impossible to determine which element had been of most benefit to her. When I asked her whether she had any idea, her answer came without the slightest hesitation: the sessions with me. It is not from a place of ego that I write this but from a deep, deep sense of gratitude.

12

Joanna's Story

Type of cancer at our first session: breast cancer
Dominant character defence: rigid

Small in stature but big in personality—that was how Joanna struck me when I first met her. Her most striking features were her eyes. They were hidden behind a pair of round glasses and it was not that they were big, but they were wide open, as if looking forward to our meeting, to meetings in general, to life itself, to the future. Her stride was resolute, her posture erect, her approach direct and open, her handshake firm. All in all, she oozed confidence. This confidence may have developed through her job as a very successful director in the corporate world in the North of England, or there again, perhaps confidence had been a prerequisite for the job.

Her story is short and sweet. I include it here because it is uncomplicated and straightforward—very much like the woman herself, with her come-on-let's-go-for-it attitude. As client/healer we met for a single series of treatments: four appointments spread out over one week. To me, she was a classic example of how easily and fast healing can occur when the physical body, emotional release, mental attitude and spiritual faith are in alignment and only need some support or clarification for sessions to be successful.

Roughly six months before we met, Joanna had discovered a lump in her right breast, had had it examined, and discovered that it was, thankfully, a benign cyst; unfortunately (or perhaps fortunately), cancerous activity was discovered in the other breast. She underwent surgery, radiotherapy, and a follow-up consultation was scheduled with the oncologist the following week since he had suggested check-ups every six months.

Joanna's mother had passed away when she was 19 years old. Partly in response to this early loss, she had entered a convent and lived the life of a Catholic nun for many years. The structured lifestyle of a convent, with a strict daily routine, provides the perfect container for a person with a predominantly rigid defence. It provided an ideal place to suppress any emotions she was feeling.

After a while, Joanna began to find religious life too restrictive. She realized that her priorities had shifted and felt that her calling was preventing her from living a fulfilling life. Once that realization dawned, she made the decision to "jump over the wall", as the saying goes. Not only did she leave the order but she also stopped participating in any form of religion. The cancer scare had changed all that, though, and she had now renewed her strong connection with Mother Mary, in whom she found the support she needed to shoulder the burdens the illness had thrust upon her.

During the intake, Joanna disclosed that she had been sexually assaulted at 14 years old. She had never really worked on the issue therapeutically, which was evident to me when we started to work together.

Once I began to run energy through her body, I found that the right side was severely blocked; in other words, a trauma was stored there and preventing energy from flowing freely. It was impairing the right side of her immune system and exposing the entire right side of her body to illness or injury, due to the fragility of the body's energetic buffer zone (one of the functions of a healthy aura).

The right side of the body is the predominantly male side, the side of doing, thinking, activities, work, analysis, and so forth. It is also the side where people store unresolved issues with significant males in their lives such as their father, brother, ex-partner, or husband. Joanna ticked that box.

She also had a closed fifth (throat) chakra. The traumatic experience had been suppressed for decades. Not a word had come up from the depths of her traumatized sexual organs, through throat and mouth, to support trauma release. Another telling symptom of the same experience is a tight shoulder girdle. Shoulders, throat, and jaw hold onto and suppress the truth and expose these parts to psychosomatic symptoms, such as sore throat, underactive or overactive thyroid, grinding of the teeth (see also Chapter 2), and so on—symptoms I come across time and time again.

In the outside world, Joanna was a well-established career woman who performed well and was involved in a stable, long-standing, intimate relationship. Her internal world, however, showed a very different picture, symbolized by years of frequent nightmares. Decades of suppressing her innermost emotions had contributed to her becoming ill, and as a result of locking away these deeply traumatic and humiliating experiences, she was experiencing long-term stagnation of her life force.

In a nutshell, this meant that her energetic body was unable to radiate fully and her physical body was unable to absorb energies essential for the upkeep of a vibrant immune system; as a result, both bodies had become exposed to imbalances. This is the essence of disease: imbalance. Nothing more, nothing less.

Feelings of internalized, inaccessible rage were apparent in the pelvic area, where I noticed dark energies brewing during our first session, but as yet there was no outlet, no voice, and the shoulder girdle held on tightly. At the start of session two, Joanna reported that she had had no nightmares the night before. As part of the second treatment, I started to dislodge the relational cord from her second (pubic/sacral) chakra, which was still attached to and connected with the perpetrator. Suddenly the rigidly held, emotional dam burst, her vocal cords were liberated, and the fifth chakra opened. Yelling and sobbing and crying and shouting and raging for about quarter of an hour released the energetic block. The flow of energy had been reawakened on her right side, and Joanna instantly felt calm and at peace.

She told me at the beginning of session three that she'd been crying buckets after the second healing, so I worked on connecting heart and pubic/sacral chakras (fourth and second). In combination with the intense release during and after session two, all tension in her shoulders, throat, and jaw melted, and she yawned repeatedly for at least half an hour.

The yawning happens automatically when the ligaments and tendons surrounding the jaw joint let go of the habitual holding in of "inappropriate" emotions. Such yawning is like jaw yoga. In my experience, this is the most effective way of stopping the ingrained habit of grinding teeth. In Joanna's case, it was a clear sign that the emotional release was positively affecting the physical structure. At the same time, her upper body spasmed involuntarily as streamers of energy flushed the system, which was as yet unfamiliar with such a surge of energy.

When Joanna arrived for the fourth and final session, she could not keep a straight face and said that it was impossible to stop laughing and singing. Her complexion looked at least 10 years younger than when we started, which had been just five days earlier.

All of this is three years ago now. We've had no further sessions together. However, she signed up for and completed the Bodies of Light certification programme and was pure joy and fun to have as a student—bright as a bubble, light of heart, kind and compassionate towards herself as well as others, deeply questioning her inner process.

Did she manage to heal the root cause of her cancer in only four treatments? Yes is my unhesitating response. Sometimes that's all it takes, when everything comes together and falls into place to complete the jigsaw puzzle of health.

13

Josh's Story

Type of cancer at our first session: cancer of the liver
Dominant character defence: masochistic

Josh contacted me for the first time in July 2012. She looked younger than her 50 years, had a daughter of seven as well as two grown-up, independent sons (all of whom had been delivered through caesarean section), and a life expectancy of no more than six months according to the medical profession.

The liver cancer diagnosis six months ago had come as a great shock. Her biggest fear was death—not really for her own sake but for her daughter's. Under no circumstance did she want to leave the apple of her eye behind. This was mainly because her husband, the daughter's father, displayed little sense of responsibility or the maturity to raise her on his own.

Amongst the notes I made about our first session are these observations: *"Holding in – biting lower lip incessantly – husband not aware of seriousness of illness – Norwood. Joint session?"*

The "Norwood" reference points to Californian author Robin Norwood, who wrote the global best-seller *Women Who Love Too Much* in the 1980s, a book that is still relevant to millions of women, married or in relationship. The book, according to one reviewer, "Describes loving too much as a pattern of thoughts and behaviour which certain women develop as a response to problems from childhood. This book shows how unhealthy these relationships are. It features a specific programme for recovery from the disease of loving too much."

Biting the lower lip incessantly indicates a tendency (mainly in women, as I rarely see the behaviour in men) to hold back verbal expression and physically manifest it as a subconscious habit. Most of the time, the husband is unaware of this tendency on his wife's part, and nor is the woman herself. Both husband and wife develop a pattern of the woman obeying the man. She does this mainly to keep the peace, to appease him, to follow the dynamics of society's behavioural patterns over the centuries, and often because she herself is fully unaware which steps or choices she would prefer. He does this mainly because society's behavioural patterns seem to have granted him the position of the one to be obeyed, because he revels in it, and because he is often unaware that his wife might even have any of her own individual needs, desires, and wishes, or even her own identity.

These are the traits of a person with a predominantly masochistic character defence, and Josh fitted the description to a T: obedient to someone else's needs, wishes, and desires to such an extent that her own wishes, needs, and desires were put on the back burner, denied, and often no longer recognized or acknowledged as such.

"Joint session" indicates that I suggested couple counselling, either here or elsewhere. The suggestion was based upon registering how the dynamics between husband and wife had been a prime cause of Josh holding back her essence, clipping her wings and freedom of spirit, and leading to self-criticism. Her inner critic carried a harsh voice, as is often the case within a masochistic structure.

Year after year, decade after decade, a harsh inner voice gnaws at a person's insides and causes them to fester. The festering process erodes the healthy functioning of organs, partly due to an automatic restriction in breathing, and instead, toxins accumulate. Underfunctioning organs are no longer capable of excreting the toxins, so they begin to clog the digestive system, and this in turn reduces the energetic frequency in and around the affected body part. The lowering of the energetic frequency gives way to psychosomatic illness of the digestive system and organs; at this point, cancer may manifest physically, since it carries a very low frequency and can only arise in a body where the innate high frequency is being restricted.

The importance of the energetic frequencies of how we live our normal everyday life can never be emphasized enough. That's why I included microbiologist Bruce Tainio's list of energetic frequencies and what they relate to in Chapter 6.

That Josh's naturally high frequency was being restricted was obvious. Her sweetness of speech, demeanour, and attitude were striking, but her sweetness had become her downfall. Sweetness is such is a beautiful trait in people. It exhibits loving kindness, compassion, and a capacity for forgiveness towards fellow human beings and/or towards all sentient beings in their vicinity. If this quality stems directly from the essence of the person, graceful composure and communication can be the result. If not, apparent sweetness may well put a very different chain of events in motion.

Sweetness can easily function as a smiling mask of compliance to the detriment of the person herself. Compliance out of obedience may well turn into resentment, initially subconscious but most likely gradually shifting into conscious awareness. Once consciously aware, the person in question directs resentment towards themselves and not towards the ones who expect and demand that the person live up to their expectations. Overtly or covertly, they will convey the message that the person's behaviour and attitude are disappointing. Judgement from so-called near and dear ones moves into self-judgement. The entire process is steeped in resentment—resentment towards oneself, one's own actions, and a sense of failing in duties and responsibilities. Resentment towards husband, family and friends, and duties and responsibilities is, within the realm of sweetness, not allowed to be either felt or expressed. Unexpressed resentment creates guilt, simmering under the skin, which turns into anger after a while—anger directed at the self.

There we have it: unexpressed anger turned inwards is a cause of cancer, words I remember so distinctly from teachings at the Barbara Brennan School of Healing (see Chapter 3).

Anger is stored in the liver, according to Louise Hay, author of *You Can Heal Your Life*. As noted above, the liver receives less energy when it becomes clogged with stagnated, unexpressed emotion. Its energetic frequency reduces as a result and creates the perfect feeding ground for cancer cells to gather, clog together, and multiply. No longer does the liver's reduced circulation suffice to disperse unwanted cellular activity.

So it was that the seemingly innocent action of biting the lower lip gave me sufficient observational material to unravel the marital, relational pattern Josh found herself locked into.

Josh's reflections about her childhood revealed situations where rage seemed utterly justified, but she had suppressed her feelings in order to take the easy way out and keep the peace. Who expects as a child or teenager that, decades later, a life-threatening illness may result from keeping the peace within the family unit?

Her father had betrayed Josh's family by starting a parallel family, with neither family having the slightest suspicion of the double life he was leading. Once the situation became unbearable, he left to live with his new family. A long-repressed image surfaced for Josh during her second treatment: the memory of sitting at the window waiting for her father's return, day after day. He never did return. Imagine the pain the child went through, day after day.

Her mother, traumatized by the secretive goings on, passed away at a young age, when my client had only just reached 20 years old. As the result of a promise she had made to mother on her deathbed, Josh took it upon herself to be the guardian of her younger sister. Her own grief was swallowed in the process. The 24-year-old became surrogate mother to a teenager way before she was ready to fulfil such an adult task.

The impact of the second session, a double, was huge. Emotional outburst followed emotional outburst. Rage, grief, and anger burst the seams of decades of emotional imprisonment. The cancerous liver reduced in size, visibly and palpably.

As we have discussed, the liver stores anger, so the release from bottled-up feelings of rage uncorked the liver and the swollen organ leaked toxicity, which was picked up and moved as circulation increased. During the final stages of the treatment, she exclaimed with great enthusiasm how much lighter she felt, how much more space had been created in her abdominal area and around the diaphragm.

Four appointments were spent on energetic healing work and verbally unravelling traumatic childhood experiences. A clearer picture emerged for Josh herself about how she'd been conditioned into a woman who had attracted cancer. She began to keep a dream diary, learnt and practised self-observation, and organized meetings with her sister in between our meetings. The energetic work siphoned more and more toxic elements out of the liver and surrounding areas.

Discussions with her husband were sporadic. She tried to convince him of her love, to clarify his role, and asked him to consider her needs, wishes, and health more consistently. Naturally, I was never present during their conversations. The way they were reported back to me, it sounded as if Josh used the right words and phrases, but with a sweetness that would never paint the full picture of the devastating impact on her health. In between the lines, it was obvious that the pattern of her looking after him didn't change fundamentally.

Things took a turn for the worse when the couple were invited to a wedding. She asked him specifically not to abandon her during the festivities, given her state of vulnerability. On previous occasions, she'd spent time with female acquaintances whilst he and his mates had drunk themselves into oblivion, expecting her to clean up the mess afterwards. She made him promise to break the pattern. He promised unreservedly.

Needless to say, on the night, he had broken his promise, disappeared off with his mates and drank. She'd felt completely abandoned, disrespected, vulnerable, and disgusted and had asked a friend to bring her home early.

Alone in bed with her thoughts, Josh spiralled down into a maelstrom of confusion, despair, devastation, and hopelessness. All effort and energy, all investment of time and money had proven useless. Was there anything else she should have done? Was there more she should have initiated? Had she not done enough? Had she not been clear enough? All the familiar masochistic Norwood questions raised their ugly heads again and in full force. All the familiar inner insecurities once more fuelled her emotions without outlet. Internally fuming, she compared herself with a pressure cooker during that fateful night.

The blow to her well-being proved impossible to overcome, and her spirits sank. Downhearted and downtrodden, her eyes had lost all life, all spark, all joy. Laughter, present in abundance earlier on, failed to emerge. Fear and hopelessness had replaced all positivity.

Josh died less than two months later, leaving her daughter in the care of her husband, a man not worthy of being a husband to such a sweet and loving wife. Would he prove himself worthy of being a loving father to a gorgeous daughter of seven?

One question keeps lingering: Did he indirectly kill his wife by disrespecting her wishes, needs, and desires and by abandoning her, despite his promise to remain at her side during the wedding? If so, how many people have been killed by their so-called nearest and dearest whilst the cause of death is registered as terminal cancer? From the start, it was clear that Josh's cancer could be remedied, and her initial reactions to the sessions confirmed my intuitive sense.

These last three paragraphs contain harsh statements. Truth and reality can be harsh. And however truthful the statements may be, ultimately it was Josh who was unable to bring herself to break up the familiar and apparent security of the family unit. Ultimately, it was her fear and inability to escape the Norwood trap that prevented her from long-term, full-spectrum healing.

14

Julia's Story

Type of cancer at our first session: breast cancer
Dominant character defence: masochistic

Julia was a lively, 57-year-old chatterbox who was married with one son. She contacted me after she had been diagnosed with breast cancer for a third time. This time, abnormal cells had also been found in her right pectoral and intercostal muscles.

During our first meeting, it took Julia only minutes to pour out her heart's agony and childhood sorrow. Her parents had been locked in arguments and fights for years, and her mother had striven to create a split between father and daughter that proved so successful that, when he passed away, Julia hadn't been allowed to attend the funeral. Sorrow and guilt were still deeply embedded in her grieving heart.

Julia's mother had unwittingly created a perfect feeding ground for a maso-chistic defensive structure in her daughter. In order to keep the peace and make life with her mother manageable, the daughter was forced to swallow her true emotions: grief around the death of her father and anger towards her mother, who hadn't allowed her daughter to be present at his funeral and to grieve for him. Julia stored her emotions deep inside, as is typical with maso-chism.

As a retired teacher, she had time on her hands. The Church of England and its local activities occupied a fair share, along with committees and the church choir. Her decision to venture into therapeutic work was also connected to the church and included reiki, journeywork, and, this time around, travelling to Findhorn for treatments. This new direction had been prompted by a prayer. During a spell of silent contemplation Julia had heard the voice of God, she said, prompting her to take a new direction in life, and she had gone searching. God hadn't put any road signs along the way and had left her pondering which direction to take.

That first visit Julia had scheduled two sessions. She made good use of them and definitely didn't do things by half. Neither did her father, who was present in spirit throughout, standing at her right shoulder.

Obvious was the strong and rich relational heart cord between father and daughter. Whilst she grieved her dad and ranted towards her mum, the cord became brighter and brighter, shedding its burdensome baggage of decades. Father poured unconditional love into his daughter's heart, and the latter received it, initially unaware of the dynamic. After several minutes, however, she acknowledged that her heart seemed full. After I shared my observations with her, she opened both arms widely in the eternal gesture of surrendering and receptivity.

The tidal wave of emotional eruptions spurred me on to perform fifth-level (spiritual) surgery. For some reason, her movements were no hindrance to the guides fulfilling their task, although normally it is a prerequisite for both the client and my hands to remain still. The guides' blue laser lights, razor sharp and accurate, managed to separate more and more cancerous areas, cutting off their energy supplies from the surrounding tissues.

At the end of the "operation", my ESP indicated that only the right breast still contained cancerous cells; however, I didn't share observations with my client. Extrasensory perception is not a medical scan and cannot be proven. A practitioner in my position needs to take care to remain realistic and not convey too positive a message of findings that cannot be verified. At the same time, messages of hope are essential for a cancer client easily caught in downward emotional and mental spirals of negativity. Precise wording and use of phrases often feel like a tightrope balancing act: truthful, realistic, positive, and not overly positive at the same time.

Can cancer fade so quickly, you may ask? It can. When you combine the client's inner emotional, mental, and spiritual release process with the healer's physical and cellular work and the guides' immaculately accurate surgical surgery, this is exactly what can happen.

Can cancer appear just as instantly? That's rare. Normally, the onset of cancer entails a process of spiritual and emotional and mental misalignment, which gradually seeps into the physical body, manifesting itself as disease. You'll read versions of this process in other chapters.

On one occasion, cancer appeared within a few days, and the woman in question died as a result. She had been held up and robbed at either gunpoint or knifepoint in broad daylight on the street of our local town, which was unheard of in our rather sedate and safe area. A friend asked me to see her right away, which I did the next day by moving some appointments around.

The impact of her trauma was huge and made her shudder, stutter, tremble, and shake throughout the session. She let go of a lot, but a strong basic, existential fear was still apparent in her first chakra (rootedness and the will to live in the physical world in a physical body). It showed itself as a dark mass—sticky, gooey, and reluctant to be removed. We agreed to meet again the following week. The meeting never took place. Within days of our treatment she was dead.

The autopsy showed an abnormally aggressive spread of cancerous cells all over her body. The robber had not merely robbed her but also, indirectly, killed her. He escaped conviction for murder because it could not be proven scientifically that she had died as the result of the violent holdup.

Similarly, in Julia's case, the reason for the disappearance of her cancer could not be proven scientifically, as this third time she had decided not to undergo any medical tests or treatments. However, at the end of a treatment or series of treatments, if a client feels lighter (both in the sense of less weighted down and less dark in energies), why should it not be possible that the cancer's grip on her body has been lessened or removed altogether? I always ask the client to remain open to all possibilities, and I ask the same of you.

My second and last session with Julia that week followed a similar pattern. She literally spat out her resentment towards her mother. A plastic bowl is always close at hand to encourage clients not to hold back and hold anything in that no longer serves them. Towards the end of our session, only traces of cancer were still visible in the right breast, and Julia and her husband travelled back down south.

It wasn't until eight months later that Julia and I met again. Her right arm hurt, and a tumour the size of a tennis ball had established itself in her right breast. She had embarked on an inner journey by beginning to admit that she didn't like her mother and never had liked her, quite something to admit for somebody with a predominantly masochistic defence. During her childhood, her mother had filled her with fear, and for years she'd been exposed to rows, abuse, and smacking on an almost daily basis. How the ongoing ordeals had impacted her body became fully clear to her.

She'd taken the initiative to write all pain, injury, and fear out of her body and into poetry, birthing one poem after another with titles that all featured a variant of "The Girl, Who . . .". Also, due to God's prompting her to embark upon new directions, the parish Julia was attached to felt unsatisfactory. Texts about Mary Magdalene, the Rosicrucian Order, Theresa of France, and the like became her focus.

Whilst visiting neighbouring churches, she had crossed paths with a man called Martin. In him she found a man with whom she could discuss all of the above, and both questioned their beliefs within the dogmatic establishment they had been dedicated to for large parts of their lives. The pair became a sounding board for each other, and a meaningful, platonic friendship ensued. Julia found support for her newly discovered self and for searching new directions. Similar support had been lacking in her previous community, where eyebrows had been raised once she'd touched on sensitive subjects, questioning and challenging institution, belief, and religion. In addition, music proved a joint passion for Martin and Julia, and he persuaded her to start a choir in a Unitarian Church nearby.

With Julia's emphasis shifting from childhood and family dynamics to diversity of religion, the treatments followed suit. Traumas from previous incarnations, previous lifetimes, surfaced unexpectedly, focused on the theme of religion: religious persecutions and abuse of rank in religious orders. Energetically, Julia excreted darkness and dark forces that were reminiscent of the medieval paintings of Hieronymus Bosch and bordered on exorcism.

Over a period of five weeks, we spent the same number of treatments on these subjects. The last sentence in my file at the end of this sequence states: "*Julia is coming home more and more.*" Once again, cancer was retreating visibly.

Then things took a turn for the worse. When Julia returned six weeks later, she had a lot to report and was close to overwhelm and breaking point.

First, her husband had lost his job three weeks earlier. He'd fallen apart and left his wife to pick up the pieces.

Second, as a result of the above, Julia had applied for a job at the local educational council and was likely to get it. She'd felt pressurized into applying, and part of her resented her fate, having to sacrifice a huge chunk of her precious time, which was dedicated to her healing journey.

Third, her sister-in-law had died of cancer.

Fourth, an old dear friend had reappeared on the scene out of the blue. Previous tender feelings for each other had been rekindled. They'd made love, despite the fact that Julia had lost interest in all sexual activity eight years previously. A breast cancer procedure had brought on a difficult period of increased self-judgement. Filled with pride and oozing satisfaction, she mentioned how she had reached 12 orgasms during two days with him in a hotel somewhere.

It wasn't her only source of oozing. Her cancerous breast had done the same for a few weeks now. She reported how the tissues in her breast had constantly changed texture. They had hardened and softened and hardened, oozed, and stopped oozing, and oozed again, depending on her emotional state.

This undeniable symptom had brought about a fifth turnaround: she had consulted a medical doctor. Her GP had prescribed antibiotics and urgently recommended mastectomy to prevent a further spreading of cancerous cells. Julia refused, obviously. The unexpected budding love affair and sexual ecstasy took precedence over what she saw as medical overcautiousness and exaggeration. By no means did the two sessions that week suffice to take stock as well as heal and repair the damage inflicted by a tremendously overpowering inner confusion.

A month later, the affair continued and blossomed. Again, we had two sessions scheduled. Strong emotional release was followed by fifth-level spiritual surgery and the tumour in her breast shrank considerably. Love seemed to heal, so Julia went on a quest for love.

In the therapeutic board game The Transformation Game, developed in the Findhorn Community in 1976, one of the Insight cards reads: "There is no force in all of creation greater than the healing power of love." On her search for new directions, Julia kept quoting the phrase, finding support in its powerful significance. Julia had found love in her life, in a man as well as in quotes, books, and a different mindset.

Fast-forward another three months, and Julia had decided that she could no longer justify playing the cheating game on her loyal husband and had confessed the truth.

She again booked a couple of treatments, and it quickly became apparent that her heart was torn. Relational cords were entangled, blocking the pure flow of love into the heart chakra, thereby preventing the surrounding physical area from absorbing the necessary energies to heal. Loyalty battled with a rekindling of love and romance and left my client in turmoil. Guilt ripped her heart apart—guilt over her devastated husband and guilt over the sense of adventure she felt with her new man and their possible prospects.

Her breast oozed to such a degree that a decaying smell surrounded her. Julia had refrained from any further medical consultations and intervention of any kind. During the first treatment, clouds of dark energies lifted off her breast, and the tissue softened to the touch and the leaking lessened.

I was under no illusion that treatments of this kind would save her breast. The news didn't shock or surprise her. It didn't, however, change her mind about consulting her GP a second time. At the beginning of her second treatment, she reported how the breast had swollen like a balloon again during and after a telephone conversation with her husband. Guilt literally tore on her heartstrings. Guilt prevented any possibility of healing.

Six months later, she came for one last time for a session. She had reunited with her husband, who accompanied her, and had been fully forgiven by him. All he wanted was for her to recover.

Recovery didn't happen. Morphine eased her pain. The breast had deteriorated rapidly. She regretted nothing of the previous months' twists and turns and prepared for death. She was at peace, including her heart, glad that deeply loving experiences had filled the final stages of her life. She had loved and known she had been loved. She still loved and knew she was still being loved. That knowledge eased her transition in the end.

Several months after her passing, an e-mail arrived from her husband, filled with gratitude. In it, he asked if he could visit me with his son, whom I'd never met, as they wanted to embark on a kind of pilgrimage, following in the footsteps of the wife and mother, to help deepen the grieving process.

During our meeting, the husband asked no probing questions and expressed only gratitude. Father and son spent a considerable amount of time in the treatment room, undisturbed in their grief. The father cried openly whilst the son fought his tears back. It was a touching meeting—a true honouring of Julia and her courageous journey, which finished by instilling peace in the hearts of everyone involved in her life and death.

15

Mem's Story

Type of cancer at our first session: cancer of the oesophagus
Dominant character defence: masochistic

At the beginning of December 2012, I visited my mother (*mem* is the Frisian word for mother). It was to be a routine visit, just like others I made once or twice a year, flying from Scotland to The Netherlands, prior to combining work and pleasure at the Costa del Sol in Spain with a friend. It did not turn out that way, unfortunately.

Earlier that year, she had got everyone together for a big party to celebrate her 80th birthday. A strong woman and very much a matriarch at heart, she'd revelled in gathering the family together and being the centre of attention. The event had fulfilled a purpose for her children, nieces and nephews, and other members of the clan, but Mem seemed to have a greater purpose in bringing us together—it felt like she saw the party as the final gathering during her lifetime. I had the impression that she saw this feast as a family reunion, her final task, after which she could hand over the baton.

She had planned and organized the event down to the last detail, from the location to the caterers, and sent out invitations six months ahead of time so we had the date in our calendars. The sun was shining, service and food were excellent, and except for three relatives who were abroad at the time, everyone was there, in good spirits and bearing gifts. She beamed all day and chatted with everyone, catching up on everyone's lives, even those she hadn't seen in decades. She was in her element, deservedly so, and lapped up the attention.

All of her life she'd been in robust health, except for an episode during her 78th year, when a hospital-induced infection had brought her to death's door. She recuperated well enough to swim in the sea off Findhorn beach when she visited me for the second and last time the following year.

That December, Mem, my sister and her partner, and I went out for a meal at a beautifully refurbished restaurant in the old colonial style called Paul Kruger in the town of Heerenveen. The restaurant is named after the founder of Kruger National Park in South Africa, who had lived in the building at one time.

Mem was having a great time until a coughing attack rudely interrupted the atmosphere. She had suffered similar attacks during mealtimes on several occasions in previous weeks, and had consulted her GP, who had scheduled tests and scans the following week, when I planned on being in Spain. Whilst there, I received the message that she'd been diagnosed with cancer of the oesophagus. All Spanish activities were cancelled, flights rescheduled, and within two days I was at her side.

As could be expected, her attitude was pretty down to earth. The oncologist had recommended a PET scan to locate the tumour more precisely and to get a clearer picture of its size. After that, if size and location allowed, surgery might be an option. If the tumour proved to be too large, chemo and/ or radiotherapy might be able to reduce its volume and thus its impact on the surrounding tissues and make an operation possible.

The standard procedure was explained, as well as possible side effects. All medical staff had been very pleasant, patient, and she was grateful for their humane approach, clarifying that ultimately the choice of how and when to proceed would be hers and hers alone. That security gave a certain peace of mind amidst diagnostic turmoil.

Her quiet existence in the village, where she'd lived for 40 years with many friends around her, had been shattered. All of a sudden the focus changed—the focus of activities and conversations with her three children and wider family and friends; the focus of time in relation to GP and hospital appointments and life expectancy; the focus of priorities, now shifting to managing ill health and from a life of relative limitlessness to a life of limitations. I spent 10 days with her, including my birthday and Christmas, then I had to return to Scotland and my full diary.

Never before had I treated a close relative, and I, as her son, perceived the healing sessions as a big honour. She benefited noticeably and mentioned how she felt more breathing space after our second one. Despite this positivity and her openness and surrendering to what was for her a hocus-pocus kind of approach, something kept telling me that she knew deep within that her time on Earth had reached its final stages.

In our discussions, she often referred to dying—of not wanting to suffer prolonged agony; of wanting to die peacefully in her own home surrounded by her three children and not in the impersonal atmosphere of a hospice or care home; of not wanting to burden her children, friends, or family for any length of time; of not wanting to lose her dignity or her marbles. In a nutshell, she set the intention to die in good health.

Each time she had to go to hospital for tests, a scan, and once for a dose of radiotherapy, my sister drove her there and back, and with each appointment,

Mem's nervousness increased. In particular, her first radiotherapy treatment took its toll, both before and after the appointment. It didn't take place in her local hospital, which felt more familiar, but in the capital, and the fact, that the Dutch healthcare system provided transport there and back by taxi didn't compensate for the upheaval.

Her ability to eat and swallow improved, but for such a short period of time, she concluded that it wasn't worth the overall upset in her quiet life to continue the treatments. Besides that, it had been made clear that radiotherapy would not cure the cancer but just give her more time whilst simultaneously decreasing her life's quality.

When the oncologist suggested six treatments she reacted very assertively. Mem thanked the man for his good intentions but explained how travelling, side effects, fear, and tension felt too big a price to pay when death was imminent and neither a cure nor long-term improvement of life's quality lay within the realm of possibilities.

Mem had made up her mind. First, she discussed matters with her three children, and when she encountered no objections and only understanding from us, she asked the GP whether she would be happy to assist in active euthanasia. A patient's right to die in a manner and time of their choosing had been legalized in The Netherlands several years earlier, so both women agreed and procedures commenced.

Legal requirements were to be followed to the letter. A report was needed from her medical doctor stating that my mother had made the decision herself whilst still possessing the mental capacity to do so. A report was needed from an independent medical doctor to diagnose the illness and to conclude it to be incurable. Behind the scenes, both medical reports had to be forwarded to a judicial committee. Also, during the final week, the GP was legally obliged to pay a home visit on four consecutive days to check whether the applicant's wish was consistent.

Once all legal requirements had been fulfilled, a time and date could be agreed. On Tuesday, 3 July 2012 at 1500 hours, the GP's diary showed a free slot, so a date was set—a diary had decided when Mem was going to pass on, breathing her final breath.

A date of death to be decided by a doctor's diary sounds cold, efficient, and impersonal. It was, but more importantly, it gave the applicant, in this case my mother, peace of mind. She knew when her suffering would end. She knew that all children were going to be present during her final moments, which had been a source of worry, especially with me living overseas. A vote by the Dutch government to approve euthanasia as an option to end a person's life in the end provided my mother with peace of mind.

On Monday, 2 July, I flew from Inverness to Amsterdam and boarded the first available intercity train to Friesland. Once seated, I'd rung her number for the last time. My sister answered and told her of my arrival in The Netherlands. I heard her sigh with relief. A plane engine had exploded in front of my very eyes when I'd travelled to her 80th birthday the previous July, and while disaster had been averted, she had felt tense about me flying since then.

When I arrived, she cried with joy and grief and held onto me, literally, for dear life. Obviously she felt tense. Obviously she felt afraid. Obviously we touched on the subject of her impending death. No more than that, however. For my mother, death was a *fait accompli,* not to be avoided and only, fortunately, to be speeded up by her decision. With less than 24 hours to live, she maintained her matter-of-fact attitude—so much so that when my sister had told her earlier that afternoon that she intended to bring a pot of soup on that day for all to share, Mem had said, with her typical Dutch humour, "There's no need to make a lot, because I won't be eating any more."

What we did discuss once more were the options and offers from oncologists and radiologists that she had declined in the leadup to her decision. They would only have prolonged and worsened her agony, and side effects would have kicked in, including most likely nausea, fatigue, and hair loss. Combined with her ever-waning energy levels, she foresaw months, if not years, of suffering and dependence on both the caring professions and her three children.

It felt as if she was asking her youngest son for a final confirmation that her choice had been the right one. Of course she was aware of my work with terminally ill people, and my experience and expertise seemed to give her final permission to go ahead. During the last several years, she was aware of my ease in discussing upsetting or painful subjects and had made use of it on several occasions. Such was the case this time, when it felt even more of a privilege than previous occasions.

The TV showed a football match that evening. We watched it together. What had once held her attention throughout the full 90 minutes now lulled her to sleep. She watched, made the occasional comment, dozed, and drifted out of her body. Unbeknownst to her, she made trial runs for what lay ahead. Trial runs support the transition of life from the physical body into death and the realms beyond—to me, an indication that peace of mind had the upper hand over fear. Observing my mother's preparation for the transition increased my own inner peace, both regarding her death and her choice of euthanasia.

Her death could not come soon enough. When her attention span reached less than a football match and when a novel no longer captivated her and when the knitting she always had on the go had become too much of a bother, then life had become an unsatisfactory burden, a drag. This state of affairs was underscored when she had a spell of diarrhoea later on, and the role of mother and child was now reversed. Naturally, she struggled with being the one who needed looking after, who had entered a state of dependency, who had made a mess, leaving it for her youngest son to clean up after her. How degrading and humiliating for this strong woman who had remained independent till the very end.

I stayed up late that evening. It was just as well, as her last night was a restless one. A few times she resurfaced, sat, and watched some TV with me. The tension was palpable. It felt like the night before a journey. Which it was—a big journey, by far the biggest and most important journey of her life.

She asked whether I thought a convict on death row might experience similar feelings. I answered that I didn't think so. She had made up her own mind, whereas on death row, death and its timing were up to a court, a judge, and a jury. The convicted person might well struggle with a bad conscience and regrets as they finally faced what was a self-imposed situation, but this was not the case with her. She nodded as her only reply. The message had sunk in.

Once she stayed in bed for over an hour and her breathing had become deep, bordering on snoring, letting me know that she'd fallen asleep. I went upstairs to the attic room. It was 2 a.m.

I woke up just after 7 a.m., got up, drank a pint of water, and went for a run, an almost daily ritual that I keep up wherever I am. On the way back, my nose caught the sweet smell of honeysuckle, and I stopped and picked a bunch of the delicate twigs. When I was a little boy, I had often brought her flowers from the wild. This was that little boy's last chance to do that for his mother, and one not to be missed. It touched Mem in the way I had hoped it would. The flowers remained next to her bed for the rest of the day, for the rest of her life.

Such precious moments shared between mother and son. Would we have been able to share the same precious moments if she had arrived at death's door with a significantly reduced quality of life? If she had decided to follow the advice of the medical profession? If there had been no other option than to follow medical procedures? If there was no legal solution called euthanasia? I doubt it.

As I write this chapter describing the end of Mem's life and our final hours together, I find myself on Pipa beach in Brazil, after last weekend scattering the ashes of both parents. My mother's chosen, empowered path has, deep in my heart, convinced me that prolonging life through debilitating medical interventions creates unnecessary suffering. I didn't really need convincing.

No cat lover would put his cat through similar prolonged agony. No dog lover would put his dog through similar prolonged agony. In all countries, with the exception of Switzerland and The Netherlands at the time of writing, children are forced to put their parents through prolonged agony.

16

Naomi's Story

Type of cancer at our first session: cancer of the ovary, liver, and bowel
Dominant character defence: schizoid

N aomi was the first client with whom I journeyed intensely after her cancer diagnosis, with whom I built a strong and mutually meaningful professional relationship, and who is no longer alive. Our 20 sessions spanned two years and four months.

She was 21 years old when we first met, and accompanied by her mother. Because mother and daughter chose to stay in the bed-and-breakfast we offer in our home that first week, I had a chance to experience their dynamics up close. As is often the case, the mother showed more fear, panic, and neediness than her daughter.

Naomi's parents were divorced. She and her mother lived together overseas, whilst her father lived in England with his new partner and children. Communication between the parents was troublesome to say the least but was pretty trouble free between father, daughter, and his new family.

The previous year, Naomi had visited her doctor, complaining of stomach pains. A cyst had been discovered on her left ovary, and the ovary had been removed as a precautionary measure. Despite this, she'd recently been diagnosed with active cancer in her right ovary, liver, and bowel. The NHS in the UK offered her management through chemotherapy, basically an extension of life, but no cure, and when I saw her, she had just finished three weeks of chemo in her home country.

When a person displays a predominantly schizoid defence system, the connection to the physical world and the first (root) chakra are weakened to some extent. In energetic terms, this means a reduction in energetic flow and absorption of vital life energy in the pelvic region. It was little wonder my client's presenting complaint originated in this part of her body.

During her parents' divorce, Naomi's life had been severely disrupted, uprooted actually. Her father had remarried and had more children with his new partner, and her mother had more or less fled overseas with her daughter. For several years, Naomi's bond with her father had been strained, but he had again opened up to Naomi and was being more cooperative.

This young woman worried about her mother, and it was obvious that the mother/daughter role had been reversed. She had not uttered a word about the immense pain and rage towards both parents the situation had forced upon her, but her anger had turned inward (see Chapter 3) and corroded (see Chapter 2). She came across as headstrong, a tough cookie, during our first treatment, and it was clear that her emotions had been well and truly locked away.

Just under a week later, we began the second of the series of six treatments in total over two consecutive weeks. The oncologist had suggested that, three weeks later, he would remove her ovary, uterus, part of the liver, and free up the bladder from the intrusion of cancerous growths. Naomi didn't fancy the idea at all and was committed to live and eventually fulfil her dream of giving birth to five children.

During this second treatment, she was tired after chemo and still experiencing slight abdominal pain at the beginning of the session. Maybe tiredness weakened her defences because in no time at all, she had dropped the "I feel fine and everything is fine" mask of the previous week. She allowed herself to be held, sobbed uncontrollably, and bravely admitted that she'd rather go through the week of healings without her mother present.

This second session signalled a turning point. Energetically, we ventured into the trauma locked into her heart chakra, which allowed her to let go of the anger that had been stored in her body for years. She surrendered completely to the erupting waves of emotions—yelling, shaking, and banging with her fists on the treatment table. After the waves had subsided, she was left cocooned in the all-protective light of her guardian angel, and the spaces her release had created were filled with the all-loving, compassionate vibration of forgiveness and serenity of Christ. Naomi sensed the presence of both and felt bathed in bliss.

The third treatment revealed the deep impact of that second session on her well-being. Her energies were lighter, and she felt more positive than ever before, and I judged it the right time to start fifth-level spiritual surgery.

Two light beings entered to offer assistance. To my intuitive sense, they appeared to personify Saint Francis of Assisi and his female counterpart Clara. When I told Naomi, she burst into tears and said that she'd always wanted to live in Assisi, Italy. Her intention combined with my ESP took me by surprise. The accuracy of my revelation blew her away and increased her faith in the joint journey we had embarked upon.

Cancer now felt as if it was retreating, as I wrote in my notes. The young woman wished to embark on a journey of faith and follow her spiritual calling as is often the case with a person with schizoid tendencies.

Sessions four and five formed a double treatment. Verbal therapeutic work, mainly concerning Naomi's dynamics with her parents, preceded the energetic healing, during which time she was distracted by pain and pressure in the lower abdomen. To me, ovary, uterus, and abdomen felt lighter, if not fully light, and practically cancer free. Traces of cancer might still have lingered, but certainly no longer of a life-threatening nature. I didn't inform Naomi of my perception as I didn't want to get her hopes up about a positive outcome using just my HSP as a guide.

Just over a month later we met again for four treatments scheduled over a four-week period while Naomi stayed in private accommodation in the wider Findhorn community. Medically, her veins were now refusing to accept the insertion of needles, indicating that her physical self refused further chemo. Scan results had also confirmed that all cancer had been cleared. This was positive news considering that her initial medical prognosis had been terminal cancer with only the possibility of postponing death via chemotherapy.

Despite her clear scans, Naomi was very upset with me. As her body detoxed, her skin had broken out in spots all over, excreting dying cancerous cells. Her symptoms presented a phenomenon I have often come across. It appears that once cancer no longer has a reason for remaining physically active, the dying cancerous cells need to go somewhere (see Chapter 8). After a series of treatments, clients frequently report symptoms such as diarrhoea, breaking out in spots, strong-smelling urine, and night sweats. To me the process of actual excretion of dead cancer cells is physical proof that healing is being integrated on all possible levels. In Naomi's case, with the addition of juicing, detox footbaths, and a change in diet, her skin returned to normal within a couple of days.

During these four weeks, her parents had engaged in a serious argument about financial arrangements. Instantly, Naomi's liver responded by indicating the onset of renewed cancerous activity. She sensed how energetic pressure drained away from the organ during the clearing treatment, and we concluded that love was her biggest asset in healing and remaining healthy. Experiencing how quickly the resurfacing of an old, illness-inducing pattern can trigger recurrence of a disease proved to be a stark life lesson for my client. To counteract any illness in future, she set a strong intention to not waver from love.

With that promise to herself she moved back overseas, to live with her mother and her aunt, in whose house she would be living. She was in great shape and filled with an incredible sense of gratitude for all life could offer her and for all she could offer life.

Almost a year later Naomi returned to see me in Scotland. Her time with her mother and aunt had been horrific. Her self-promise of love had been crushed out of her by both adults, and once again rage had been internalized. She had moved to Assisi a couple of months before arriving on my doorstep in order to fulfil a lifelong wish to follow in the footsteps of Saint Francis and Clara, and it was here that a scan had shown a 6-centimetre tumour around her right ovary and two tumours in her bladder and uterus of almost 2 centimetres each.

Again, we cleared the emotional baggage, and again, Naomi managed to be filled with the light of Christ, Saint Francis, and Clara. During our third and final session, she was pain free and the biggest of the three tumours, which had been clearly palpable before, could no longer be traced. Again, the next month's scan proved all cancer to have vanished. Again, the medical profession was baffled and found itself unable to explain the recovery.

It was at the end of that fourth session that Naomi spontaneously burst out crying—tears of gratitude for her health being restored. Mainly, though, tears of gratitude for having had cancer and for cancer having taught her vital life lessons ordinary life could never have taught her with such clarity.

Fourteen months after this episode (we didn't meet during the interim period), the cryptic notes in Naomi's client file stated the following:

Only eating yoghurts. Tumour around colon and bladder. Morphine and anti-sickness medication. Transition time: fully healing or pass over, but intention is to live long and publish her story of healing. Mum and family abroad filled with fear. N. staying with dad and family: OK. Last scan February: not operable and calcifying—half a year to live. Felt a few times at death's door. Bulk of cancer in lower pelvis, incl. bowel and bladder—stagnating digestion. Liver slightly affected. Main issue: mum. Family in England healed—haven for N. to heal. Healing: deep release from tumour and rage. Afterwards light. Christ present.

The next day's notes:

Feels as if calcified tumour around colon releases. N. already eaten some tatties!!!!! Tummy rumbling continuously, and N. feeling debris moving up and out.

My notes two days later:

Ate big meal of real food!!!!! First in months. Needs to release toxic care for mum. Voice: "You are deeply loved" and surrendering into love. Emotions with me reiterating it. Feels largely clear towards the end.

Two months later the request came for me to visit her in a hospice in England, where she'd been admitted. By that time, tumours had spread all over Naomi's abdomen, colon, and duodenum. She was only taking in liquid. Even that did rarely pass, and her body was unable to take any of it in, let alone digest it. Her seventh (crown) chakra, the gateway to the realm of spirit and higher consciousness, was wide open. Her first (root) chakra, the energetic connection to Earth and earthly incarnation, was tiny and in the process of dissolving. The latter can indicate the beginning of a client's dying process.

The family had turned her room into an amazingly tranquil sanctuary, with statues of many deities, candles, incense, and chanting CDs playing almost constantly—a piece of Heaven on Earth, aiming to ease the transition. All family members came and went in deep, honouring respect and sadness.

Still, on her deathbed, Naomi reminded everyone to look after her mum. Still, on her deathbed, she was incapable of reversing roles and allowing herself to be the daughter of her mother. She died peacefully, surrounded by the ones she wished to be present.

A couple of months later, I received a phone call from her stepmum. Because of me having been able to support Naomi twice in eradicating all cancer, the stepmum (herself a medical doctor by profession) wondered why healing had not been possible a third time around.

My answer: "She was unable to stop caring for her mum at her own expense and reverse the roles back to the original, healthy mother/daughter relationship."

Stepmum's reply: "Interesting you should say that. About a month before she died, her dad had a long discussion with Naomi about her mum and told her plainly that if this is what she really thought, why not tell mum." Naomi's answer had been: "I can't tell her that, Dad. I'd rather die."

Ultimately, it was Naomi's choice to protect her mother until her dying breath. No doctor, healer, or oncologist can work against an intention held with such conviction.

17

Patricia's Story

Type of cancer at our first session: breast cancer
Dominant character defence: masochistic and schizoid combined

Chatty, bubbly, lively, and beautiful—these were my initial impressions when Patricia exited her rented car. She had travelled from overseas, and a slight clumsiness with the seatbelt and the closing of the door indicated that she was not that used to driving a British car.

She exuded an attitude of ease and a carefree life, able to face all manner of challenges life threw in her direction. Automatically on meeting such a positive-minded person, despite them facing a considerable health scare, I question whether their attitude is authentic or whether it is a facade, a mask. If the latter proves to be the case, then how far, to what extent, how frequently, and under what circumstances does the person apply the facade that all is well. And what remains hidden beneath the mask? These first impressions hinted at a predominantly masochistic defence.

Of course, I did not share my inner musings with Patricia. These types of observations are stored somewhere in the back of my mind to be utilized at a later stage, depending on what the client brings to the sessions.

Patricia's presenting complaint was stage 2 cancer of the left breast. The disorder had been diagnosed about six months before our first meeting. In the meantime, she'd undergone surgery and radiation. The stage 2 diagnosis meant that the cancer was at high risk of returning and spreading in spite of the medical interventions, so chemotherapy had been recommended. Decisive as she was, Patricia had embarked on her own journey by consulting a naturopath, a homeopath, a herbalist, and an iridologist.

For her, the inner journey really took off during a series of life coaching sessions. Her so-called feminine wound began to surface and gave Patricia the push she needed to connect with her inner and outer worlds, with the aim of healing the root cause of her breast cancer. She had not yet fully made up her mind, but was strongly considering going ahead with the chemo and using herbal and homeopathic remedies to reduce the side effects of the treatments.

On arrival, Patricia still suffered post-operative discomforts in her left armpit. We had three treatments planned that week. During the first session,

I restructured her first (root) chakra to boost her overall immune system, after which I did the same with her left breast and armpit. Encouragingly, her pains had vanished by the beginning of session two. This type of tangible positive result offers immediate hope that the work the client and I will be doing together will bear fruit. It was a very encouraging start.

Patricia's first (root) chakra seemed not to be as deeply rooted in the earth as one might expect, and the tip of the chakra seemed not fully connected to the energetic anatomy of her system, which consists of seven major chakras and the interconnecting channel, the Vertical Power Current. In other words, if my ESP was painting an accurate picture, there was a disconnection between Patricia as incarnated being and the earth upon which she had incarnated. When this is the case, the body's immune system suffers because it is energized (or not, as was the case with Patricia) by the root chakra.

At the beginning of session two, I asked whether she knew anything about her birth or her mother when she'd been pregnant with her. As described in an earlier chapter, if the foetus or baby has experienced a traumatic pregnancy or birth, the first, subconscious, imprint on the infant's being is that life in the physical realm is traumatic, scary, and frightening. As a result, the infant is being conditioned into creating or maintaining a loose or noncommittal connection with the earth and their own physical incarnation.

One of the main energetic defensive patterns due to this schizoid defence structure is an underdeveloped root chakra. This can lead to an equally under-developed immune system. Had the foetus and/or the baby Patricia faced an early trauma?

Her reply to my question spoke volumes. She'd been born prematurely, that is, before the full term of the pregnancy had been completed, and although it was a natural birth, it had been medically induced. The reason why her mother had chosen or had been recommended to follow this rather drastic medical procedure was unknown, and her mother may well have had no choice in the matter. More often than not, a baby's traumatic birth is not the mother's fault.

During the writing of this book, I spoke to a friend from Dumfries & Galloway in southern Scotland about this book and its theme of a predom-inantly psychosomatic cause of cancer. She questioned my opinion. A four-year-old girl in her neighbourhood had just been diagnosed with cancer of both kidneys. How could such a wee lassie have experienced such severe stress or tension that it brought on the illness, my friend queried?

I explained the theories of Wilhelm Reich's schizoid defence and how a traumatic birth can undermine the healthy development of the first chakra, which is responsible for energizing the immune system as well as the kidneys and adrenal glands. I explained that the adrenal glands produce the hormone adrenaline, which is activated during a fear response, and the kidneys, which sit directly below the adrenals, are the organs associated with fear. On hearing that, my friend reacted with surprise. She explained that the couple had tried for a baby for years, had had a miscarriage about a year earlier, and that the wee lassie had been the result of IVF treatment.

Imagine the stress both parents had faced during the second pregnancy, the one that led to the birth of the little girl in question. Would the mother be able to give birth this time? Would they face yet another huge disappointment? In the mother's mind, she might well have wondered whether she had failed in motherhood during the first pregnancy. What kind of stress and tension did the mother put herself under in order to finally give birth to a healthy baby? The foetus in the womb grows inside a container of tension. How can this tension not affect the unborn baby? Stress inside the womb may well have been the main cause of cancer of the kidneys in the girl, only four years of age.

In Patricia's case, a premature, artificially induced birth may well be nothing more than a routine job for the medical profession and not at all feel like a trauma for the mother, but for the infant it can be a totally different experience. The natural flow of pregnancy and birth is being interrupted, and the speedy, artificial procedure can come as a shock to the baby. The entire process of birth, therefore, most likely came as something of a shock to tiny and vulnerable Patricia.

Knowing this intimate detail concerning my client's birth clarified for me that we needed to take extra care working with Patricia's first chakra. Whereas strengthening the root chakra is a pretty standard part of treating a person with cancer, because of the sometimes life-threatening condition, in Patricia's case I needed to give it extra attention.

Two deeply buried emotions are prevalent for a person with a schizoid past, namely fear and rage. The subconsciously stored fear was due to the medical intervention prior to Patricia's birth. The baby can perceive the intervention as a life-threatening experience because, at that stage, all the infant experiences is life itself. If life itself is under threat, fear turns into a predominant emotional charge.

The subconsciously stored rage can be explained: coming from the realm of light in between lives (if incarnational theories can be believed, which I do), the infant feels subconsciously trapped in an unsafe, life-threatening physical body. It feels like a harsh existence compared with the realm of light.

The infant has no choice in the matter of incarnation and can easily feel rage about having been forced to leave the light against its will to incarnate physically. This emotional charge lies dormant, subconsciously stored; therefore, a person with a schizoid character defence often displays a life pattern of seemingly unfounded fearful responses and unreasonable attacks of rage with a tendency to dissociate from daily reality.

Patricia ticked all of the above boxes. She disclosed at the beginning of the second session that she recalled barely any childhood memories (dissociation from reality is a typical schizoid tendency). One series of events she did remember vividly, though, was that she hid frequently in the toilets at school, for no apparent reason.

'For no apparent reason', according to the adult woman sitting opposite me, but schoolgirl Patricia no doubt will have had her reasons for hiding and likely experienced some level of fear at that time. Why else hide? Who or what was she hiding from? Who or what had she perceived as a threat? We never got to the bottom of little Patricia's inner turmoil.

Whatever her answer may have been, often these kinds of dynamics are being influenced by the relationship between the individual and a certain person or certain people in the direct social environment. Energetic relational cords between the various chakras of the various individuals store significant dynamics, the pleasant ones as well as the unpleasant ones. Therefore I explored relational cords during our third session. The notes in her file describe the following:

Through working with her cords, chakra three opened wider and deeper than before. Lots of sadness and anger surfaced and was expressed, especially from throat and jaws, through screaming incessantly. Fists pounded the couch in unbridled rage.

I remember that after the cathartic outburst my client's eyes shone brighter, her smile had widened, and the jaw joint released years of tight clenching, her chest felt and looked freer, allowing for a more liberated breath, and it seemed as if the cancerous activity withdrew somewhat.

Patricia flew back home. She returned just over a month later and had aged visibly. The first chemo treatment had just been and gone at that point. As is often the case, my client did not show many side effects initially; however, her lips, cheeks, and chin felt numb and restricted in movement, affecting her speech slightly. Also her left arm, hand, and fingers felt numb. There was no hair loss yet. Patricia did expect to lose her hair sooner or later and displayed a pretty laissez-faire attitude towards hair loss, but she feared for her eyebrows and eyelashes falling victim to chemotherapy—that she didn't wish upon herself.

The first session was spent restructuring her root chakra and cleansing the aura in the affected areas, mainly around the upper left side of her body. Following her request, I put extra emphasis on strengthening the first level of her aura around her eyes to prevent her losing eyelashes and eyebrows. My comments in her file at the beginning of session number two read as follows:

Much better. Almost all side effects of the chemo have vanished. She looks 10 years younger than yesterday.

As I described in "Famke's Story" in my book *Cancer: A Healer's Perspective*, ridding a patient's body of the side effects of chemotherapy can indeed be that easy, that instant, and that straightforward.

Physical symptoms occur more often than not as a result of energetic blocks in a person's aura. The chemical substances within chemotherapy create energetic debris in the human energy field. If and when the aura is cleansed prior to the energetic blocks turning into physical symptoms, many side effects of chemo (if not all) can be prevented. Along similar lines, once physical symptoms have set in, as with Patricia, side effects can be reduced or remedied entirely by cleansing the aura.

Is it always necessary to consult a healer to achieve this result, you may wonder? No. There are many ways to purify one's energetic field. I often recommend spending time at the seaside, because the salty breeze is effective as an auric cleanser. Equally effective can be, for example, smudging, which entails using the smoke of smouldering sage or cedar to remove energetic debris.

Besides these anticipated distortions in her aura, Patricia was scared. Directly adjacent to where the needle of a hormone injection had penetrated her skin, she had discovered a rather sharply painful lump. When fear is already a dominant feature in a person's emotional makeup (as with Patricia's schizoid defence structure), it can take very little to ignite a new wave of fear. The slightest hint of cancer spreading or returning can change the person in question from a confident and hope-filled individual into a scared, emotional wreck.

This was most definitely the most alarmed I'd seen my client. She almost begged me to use my ESP to check whether the lump was malignant or "simply" the result of the injection possibly having touched a nerve. The piercing of the skin had been considerably more painful than on any previous occasion.

When I tuned in clairvoyantly, I didn't detect any darkness, and that is how I visually register cancer: black blobs in the aura or inside the body. As noted before, though, I don't tell my clients whether there is or is not cancer according to my ESP. As a non-medical practitioner without medical equipment available, I cannot make such a direct statement. What I said at that moment will have been along the lines of what I've just written. I told her what I saw, or rather what I didn't see, and I informed her how I usually registered cancerous growth.

However carefully and diplomatically I worded my findings, though, Patricia greedily took them for gospel and cried with relief and reassurance. It became obvious how much tension she had stored due to the seemingly innocent, albeit painful lump. It also became obvious to me how well she'd managed to cover up her tense and fearful state during the first quarter of an hour of our treatment. Once the stress had left her, she relaxed visibly. Fear had gripped her more than ever before, but so too had relief and relaxation afterwards, and she yawned repeatedly.

We spent the remaining four scheduled treatments unravelling her past. Visit number three, several weeks later, when she was now bald from the second chemo treatment, followed a similar pattern of first, removing the effects of chemo so Patricia could maintain quality of life, and second, exploring the conditioning of her childhood years.

It didn't take long for both of us to recognize that much of the smiling attitude she exhibited in daily life was indeed a mask, as I had suspected from the start. Initially, I worked with this by remaining totally in the present and reflecting back to her how brightly and seemingly upbeat she had entered the house and the healing room that first day of her second visit, and how chatty she'd come across, but how her demeanour had, on reflection, been a mask to cover up her inner emotional turmoil. Had she at that moment exhibited a pattern she found herself familiar with?

A rather long, reflective silence followed. During such moments, I pull back energetically to provide space for the client, and I quietly observe any fluctuations in their aura and chakras.

Patricia's aura contracted and became denser as she pulled into herself to create space for inner reflection. In her aura, a red blob appeared around the liver. Livers store anger/rage. Did she, knowingly or unknowingly, begin to get in touch with stored anger or rage? The aura around her pelvic region, normally dullish in colour, became more activated, as if something was brewing beneath the surface. Were deeply hidden emotions preparing to surface? What followed was an almost standard unravelling of the predominantly masochistic character defence:

Smiling as usual, Patricia recalled how she, as a little girl, had been the sunshine of the family. She'd never complained, had always agreed with virtually everything, had cared for and looked after her younger sister, and had engaged in all manner of chores without being asked.

When I asked in return who had looked after her when she was little, her answer, not unexpectedly, was: "Mainly me. I got myself up, dressed myself, got my own breakfast, and often took care of my sister in the process."

"The main question here, Patricia," I said, "is, did you do all these chores voluntarily of your own pure free will or did a hidden agenda rule your actions—the hidden agenda of wishing to act as a good girl in order to please your mum?"

Her reply came in a whisper from an adult woman there and then regressed into a little girl who became very shy with downcast eyes.

"I wanted to please my mum, but in such a way that she would pay less attention to me. I wished her to be less bothered about me. It felt as if she invaded me. She didn't give me the space I longed for, and that's why I rejected her. For quite some time I didn't even want her to touch me. What I longed for more than anything else was her genuine interest in me."

"Thank you, Patricia. That's a brave thing to admit. You wanted to please your mother in order for her to love you for who you really were, and for your mother to pay less attention to you, and for you to be acknowledged as your own person with your own identity. Something like that?"

Still with downcast eyes the little girl in an adult body nodded in silence.

As we've seen before, the woman embodied a strong schizoid character defence structure due to her premature birth. It is the most normal thing for an individual to take on the defensive pattern of two or three different character structures. One defensive pattern is often the more dominant one. When the main pattern has moved into the background for whatever reason (possibly through therapeutic work or a change in life's circumstances), another defence may well surface temporarily. Different patterns can surface within the same person, depending on social circumstances. The same individual can portray a very different persona during sporting events (possibly competing psychopathically) than in the family unit (possibly complying masochistically) or the working environment (possibly career-advancing rigidity).

Patricia's replies made clear that she'd been vying for her mother's love for the personality she felt she really embodied and for the individual she wished to grow into. My client didn't recall this tendency in herself, as such, but most likely, deep within, she will at times have resented her chores and caring for her younger sister. Obviously, in her dependent situation as a young girl, her resentment was less strong than her need for individuation, developing her own personality, and space away from her mother; therefore, resentment was being suppressed.

More often than not, people who embody a masochistic defence find it a challenge to develop an independent identity. Their development frequently goes hand in hand with a struggle for freedom. This can mean freedom from authority, freedom from parental dominance, or freedom from society's norm. When the struggle for inner liberation and acknowledgement takes many years or decades (as is most often the case), the person no longer has a true sense of their own identity and priorities.

The penny dropped for Patricia once I had explained the theory of the masochistic character defence and made the link to her own situation in her family of origin.

What about her pattern at school? She began to recall and recognize the significance of part of her behaviour as a schoolgirl (do you remember how she had been hiding in the toilets at school?) and amongst her childhood friends. Within her circle of friends, young Patricia had been a merry lassie, or a girl who had outwardly tried to portray a merry lassie, who gave most generously, despite feeling utterly lonely deep inside. Ultimately, it had been her loneliness that had made her hide in the toilets. To combat this loneliness, she'd unreservedly been kind and attentive and loyal to her friends even when they said something wrong in her opinion or rejected her.

Why such unreserved generosity of spirit? Was it her aim to seek her friends' attention by offering time, attention, and kindness straight from the heart? Was it her aim to seek their love? Was it her aim to seek friendship in order to compensate for her feelings of loneliness? It was telling when she remarked that she hadn't been able to understand how her friends had often shown little gratitude. Their tendency towards ingratitude had undermined her sense of self-worth, but it hadn't stopped her from seeking their friendship, over and over. Just imagine how much energy this longing and generosity must have taken.

Working for a governmental institution, she showed a similar pattern of feeling overly responsible. Did her lack of self-worth create that inner sense of responsibility beyond her duties in her working environment?

Gradually, more pennies dropped for Patricia about how her original family unit had conditioned her to comply with what other family members wanted or expected of a daughter and a sister without fully taking into account who she really was and what she craved. She began to realize that she hadn't lived her life according to her own priorities. Instead, her priorities had shifted according to which actions might generate the love, attention, and space, hence the safety, she longed for more than anything else. The girl, and now the woman, had lived more or less an entirely disempowered existence, surrendering her own individual power to those from whom she wished to receive what she craved.

Once my client realized how much and how frequently she had compromised to the detriment of her own needs and desires and to the detriment of her own health, anger arose in full force.

Patricia raged during two consecutive sessions. The red spot in her aura around the liver area, which I'd witnessed earlier, finally and for a short period only, became the most significant auric feature. On entering the treatment room at the beginning of these two sessions, red was the dominant colour in her energetic field. And once she allowed herself to fully express her anger, there was no holding back: anger towards her mother for her sister always having received everything she asked for and Patricia not getting her needs met; anger towards her privileged sister; anger towards her ungrateful friends; anger towards many aspects of how she had grown up and how she had been raised.

One anger-triggering issue after the other surfaced and caused Patricia to let rip physically after keeping her jaws clenched tight and withholding the expression of her emotions for decades. She banged with her fists on the couch. She kicked violently. She screamed and yelled and howled and swore. She coughed incessantly, spat, and puked. She sweated profusely.

The next day, she looked and felt exhausted. After the second of the two explosive sessions she had done little else other than rest, drink, and sleep, with the deep and dreamless sleep interrupted only by a multitude of toilet visits. Despite drinking a great deal of water, Patricia's urine remained coloured and smelly. The cells of her body were excreting copious amounts of toxicity, which had been stored for almost the entire duration of her life as a result of storing her emotional baggage and not permitting herself to live an authentic life.

It was during this treatment that she made a promise to herself to live authentically from then on, to stop betraying herself, to no longer allow others to override her boundaries, and to put herself, her well-being, and her priorities before those of the people around her. There was a clear feeling of dedication, power, and strength emanating from Patricia. She sat straighter. Her feet were planted firmly on the floor. Her eye contact was unwaveringly direct. Her voice carried more volume.

After the last treatment of her fourth visit, my file reads:

Did we achieve cancer cure at root level this week? It feels like it!. . . For the first time chakra 1 reacts very strongly during restructuring.

At the beginning of the first session of her next visit, my file reads:

Chakra 1 has remained and is now strong at the beginning of P's visit.

Encouraged by her inner shift, Patricia embarked on a deepening journey of self-discovery, self-validation, and self-respect by extending her inner work through workshops and therapy, elsewhere, as well as here at Findhorn.

She and I have reached the stage that she only contacts me on the rare occasion she needs a top-up, for a brief consultation via e-mail, or for a distant healing. Patricia has well and truly broken through her painfully restricting past. To a large extent, she has managed to shed her schizoid and masochistic character defence structures. At the time of writing, it has been almost two years since we first met, and I am in no doubt that Patricia will remain cancer-free. She is a brave woman who definitely deserves credit for what she has achieved therapeutically.

19

Pauline's Story

Type of cancer at our first session: ovarian cancer
Dominant character defence: masochistic

Out of the taxi stepped a fairly heavy-set woman, slightly stooped, with her head tilted forward, as if the world's burdens were weighing heavily on her neck and shoulders. Three times before closing the car door, she confirmed and questioned the arrangements she'd made with the driver, just to make sure he'd return her to the B&B in town after our time together.

This all played out before she noticed me standing in the doorway. As soon as she became aware of my presence, apologies poured forth from her about being early, but she couldn't help it, because the taxi had arrived about quarter of an hour too soon and therefore she couldn't keep him waiting until the appointed time, and she'd happily go for a stroll if I wasn't ready, which she could well imagine, because . . . and so on. Her hand felt clammy to the touch and the handshake weak.

A session often begins well before the client enters the treatment room because observations are not limited to these four walls. In this case, the client's posture and mannerisms were enough for me to determine that she displayed a predominantly masochistic defence. The giveaway was her heavy body, her tendency to double-check arrangements in order to "not get it wrong", and to apologize far more than necessary to get her point across.

In the treatment room, she answered my intake questions in a long-winded manner. When I asked her about her presenting complaint, she started by telling mother's story. Mum had been bedridden before death put an end to two years of agony, and Pauline had supported her mother devotedly through progressive ovarian cancer. Witnessing her mother getting weaker had a strong impact on Pauline, and afterwards, gruesome images kept haunting her. She developed the strong belief that she also would at some point in her life be faced with ovarian cancer. Sure enough, a couple of decades later, all of her suspicions were confirmed when she was diagnosed with ovarian cancer.

The medical profession might well label Pauline's illness as hereditary, as a fait accompli, as genetically stored and manifested in generational genes. In my experience and opinion this is rarely the case. Pauline had been severely traumatized by her mother's slow and painful deterioration, and the images she'd been left with became imprinted on her brain. In her mind's eye, she saw herself in her mother's place, and over time, these images settled into her aura, especially the third (mental) level. Her mentality changed her aura from a health risk–reducing buffer zone into an energetic minefield that contained the energetic template for attracting the same disease as her mother. It was an example of a self-fulfilling prophecy.

Losing sight of one's own identity, partly due to overidentifying with another person (my client overidentifying with her mother and her illness) is typical of a masochistic defence structure. The expression "to take on someone else's pain or burden" can have far-reaching consequences, as Pauline proved to her own detriment. What I tell a client at such a moment is that she and her mum are two different individuals, each walking separate, individual paths based upon a totally different life purpose for the present incarnation. The clarity of such a statement can support a client like Pauline in disentangling herself energetically from her mother's past and lay a foundation for healing her own present situation.

As we have seen, the physical world follows the energetic world or template. In other words, the physical body shapes itself in accordance with the energetic frequencies, circulation, and blocking thereof in the various layers of the aura. Out of Pauline's pre-programmed images and beliefs grew the physical manifestation of ovarian cancer. The daughter was walking in her mother's footsteps.

If my client had dealt with the illness and death of her mother in such a way that she'd been able to lay it to rest, cancer could have been prevented. The implication of this last sentence is that my client's cancer most likely had its cause in the psychological programming and not in genetic programming, as the medical profession would have it. Psychological programming, better known as conditioning, arises from a thought form, concept, or attitude that has been learned, and as such, it can be unlearned. Genetic programming, on the other hand, cannot be unlearned. It has been stored in the cells of generations of family members and can therefore feel hopeless, whereas an attitude rooted in a learned psychological mindset has the seeds of its own recovery embedded, if the person is able to change their mind.

For somebody like Pauline, reframing her thoughts offered the opportunity to move from imminent death to a state of illness, which would allow her the possibility of turning around her health, so that hopelessness becomes hopefulness. A more positive belief can make the difference between healing or not healing cancer. A client's faith in their own capacity to recover is essential to their healing journey.

In fact, despite displaying the body language of a disempowered woman, Pauline had taken giant life-changing steps, if not leaps. No sooner had her cancer been diagnosed (not an unexpected turn of events) than she started to realize how fear had been holding her back her whole life. This fear in particular related to her stepfather, a tyrant who had wedged himself between mother and daughter by continuously threatening to leave if he didn't receive preferential treatment. As soon as he had moved in, he had become abusive towards his so-called beloved and her offspring, and dominated, manipulated, and often turned to violence, physically as well as sexually, targeting both females.

After her diagnosis, Pauline had begun taking charge of her life. She had left her job and changed her diet. Her decision to consult me had been entirely her own, frowned upon but ultimately supported by her husband.

During our first session her emotions came close to the surface, and although they remained as yet unexpressed, her entire body trembled uncontrollably. There was clearly a longing for the facade that had been built up over decades to crack and for everything that had been denied a voice all of her life to come pouring out.

That voice took over in our second session the next day. Fists pounding the treatment couch, she yelled repeatedly, "How dare they! How dare they! How dare they!" The outburst released so much stored pain and rage that her entire pelvic area was aglow, including her ovaries. She looked at least 15 years younger when she left.

We met again for a couple of treatments about 10 weeks later. The previous week's scan had shown a reduction in growth of the cancer and her blood count had normalized (see Chapter 11). Her oncologist had managed to persuade her to take part in a drug experiment. Every four weeks she'd be monitored, and she would have to take the drug indefinitely, if successful; that is, for the rest of her life. Pauline didn't like this prospect and had found the courage to assert her opinion about what *she* wanted.

Simple though it might sound to the majority of readers, for Pauline to have the courage to have a different opinion from her oncologist, a person in authority, to express her view, showed a significant shift in attitude away from her previously held masochistic pattern. I made a point of sharing this observation with Pauline and complimented her on her assertiveness in order to make her aware of her inner change of attitude and encourage further developments in this direction.

After spells of intense cathartic release through shouting, coughing, spitting, crying, and trembling, Pauline was able to feel her pelvis tingling with energy, an excellent sign. Healing can only occur when energy is able to flow freely through the affected area, allowing the diseased body part to cleanse itself of energetic blockages, cancerous cells, and other sources of toxicity and to be revitalized.

At our second session, two days later, Pauline had broken out in spots, another excellent sign (see Chapter 8). I have seen this happen on several occasions, as noted earlier, and it indicates that toxins in the body have reached saturation point and are now ready to be excreted. When a body in healing mode is lifted to a higher energetic frequency, its innate intelligence leads it to want to rid itself of any stagnant energy that blocks the ability to stay on this higher frequency. The body chooses health. Each body is biologically designed to survive, and its instinct is to utilize all possible means to rid itself of dead or toxic cell material, such as strongly smelling urine, diarrhoea, sweat, or in Pauline's case, skin problems like a rash or spots.

The third series of treatments, three months later, showed a very different Pauline, one who was certainly doing her inner work. More confidence had slipped into her speech. Her posture had straightened, and she now held her shoulders and head erect. Her eyes had brightened and beamed in my direction with a sense of aliveness, whereas before, they'd been shrouded in dullness. The mental and emotional burdens carried by this masochistically programmed client had well and truly lifted, and her body had changed as a result.

Pauline's courage and commitment to her healing were not in vain. Her blood count had returned to normal, and once I sank into her tumourous area, it became clear that the growth had lost all vitality.

A lump remained and might well remain in the body for years, even the rest of her life, but without a real threat of it springing back to life as long as Pauline remained loyal to herself and her health and well-being. Sometimes such a lump of ex-tumourous matter stays in the body and functions as an indicator of how well the person is remaining on track emotionally, mentally, or spiritually.

I have often come across people whose still existent but malignant tumour hardened temporarily or began to hurt a bit when old patterns that had instigated the original cancer again reared their head. At such a moment, the body tells the person in no uncertain terms that balance has been disrupted again and inner or outer action (or both, more likely) is necessary. Under these circumstances, it is vital to listen to the body and have the awareness from previous experiences to know why the body gives the signal and act upon it. The action is the most important part of this process. Experience, knowledge, and awareness are essential ingredients, but if these are not translated into down-to-earth actions, shifts, or changes in everyday life, they remain theoretical only, without impact or result, without removal of symptoms.

Pauline was on the road to recovery from cancer through an increased self-esteem, and self-discovery. This time, she'd travelled up with her husband in their camper van. In a flash of inspiration I asked whether she drove the vehicle herself. The positive reply was followed by my question, whether she'd ever considered taking off on her own for a week or a fortnight. She hadn't. Her eyes lit up, indicating that the idea appealed to her recently discovered sense of freedom. She was fed up with her husband's life, filled with stagnation and negativity, anyway. There and then she promised herself that they'd drive home together and then she'd pack and take off.

This she did. I received a postcard from the Outer Hebrides, and much later, we met a final time just before she participated in an Experience Week at Findhorn Foundation. She had also stopped taking drugs against the oncologist's advice.

Quitting medication can be highly beneficial for some people, offering yet another step towards independence from institutions, habits, patterns, and the like. For others such a decision may well prove a step too far.

Pauline, though, had truly liberated herself and as a bonus had healed herself of her cancer.

19

Ronald's Story

Type of cancer at our first session: cancer of the stomach
Dominant character defence: schizoid combined with oral

Ronald was 63 years old when he arrived for a first session—a tall, thin, wiry man who wore glasses. A criss-cross of lines covering his entire face, and combined with slightly stooped shoulders and pensively deep-set eyes gave the impression of a life not without its fair share of worries and troubles. Married, he lived in a small satellite community in the Findhorn area.

The initial presenting complaint was reoccurring post-viral chronic fatigue syndrome (CFS). The first occurrence had been 19 years earlier, accompanied by strong flu symptoms. After two years, he managed to return to a normal working week as a self-employed psychotherapist; however, during the five years prior to our first appointment, he had, in his own words, only lived about 70 percent of his former existence and hardly saw any clients. My intake notes describe a man not given to doing things by half, with a tendency towards self-bullying behaviour. For example, he totally overdid Osho's dynamic meditation and crashed afterwards into fatigue.

Ronald received four treatments over the course of three months. There was an absence of joy in his life. He loved writing, but mainly in a self-chastising manner, where guilt had the upper hand over pleasure or fun. The main sources of guilt were related to the significant women in his life. His mother had faced a near-death experience whilst giving birth to her son, and contact with his daughters left much to be desired since, decades earlier, he had deserted his wife and children in England and joined a renowned ashram in India.

People with a schizoid wounding due to complications at birth often lack a strong connection to planet Earth and their incarnated physical bodies. In order to find the safety they crave, they frequently embark on a spiritual path, connecting through the seventh (crown) chakra with "higher" realms and ideals beyond earthly concerns. Ronald's choice to move to a spiritual community in India was an understandable option for a man who failed to find safety and satisfaction on the earthly plane.

His children had difficulty forgiving their father for abandoning them in order to pursue his own path. As a loving father and psychotherapist, he now could fully understand their stance and heaped ladles full of guilt onto his own plate, only too aware of the selfish streak that had existed in him at that stage of his life, when his daughters were still young and fragile. Basically, his plate overflowed with difficult-to-digest emotional baggage—impossible, perhaps, given such a self-imposed, heavy-handed, and guilt-laden attitude to life.

One of the character traits of an oral defence system is exactly that: selfishness linked with the innate need for feeding and being fed by external sources, because the biological feeding pattern had been interrupted soon after birth. Orally conditioned people often display a strong focus on food, diets, and making sure kitchen cupboards are full just in case a renewed interruption might follow. People with eating disorders such as bulimia and anorexia nervosa more often than not display a predominant oral character defence. Is it any wonder that Ronald had attracted cancer of the stomach, the organ directly linked with the intake of food?

After the first four sessions, we didn't meet again until two years later. He'd been briefly hospitalized a year and a half before, due to stomach trouble from having received a wrong prescription from the GP. His troubles continued. Three months before returning for treatments with me, an endoscopy had revealed active cancer cells, and a fortnight later, a scan showed a thickening of the stomach lining and an affected duodenum. Discomfort had started to set in whenever he ate or lay in bed. The oncologist had prescribed three months of chemotherapy with surgery afterwards.

Ronald and I then embarked on 20 treatments over the next 10 months. Woven through our treatments were the words his father had spoken to Ronald's eldest brother when the latter had been diagnosed with leukaemia (and later made a full recovery): "Heal your wounds, my son." Both father and brother had passed in the meantime, but his father's exhortation had inspired Ronald to embark on a journey to face his fear and internalized rage, self-chastising guilt, and to heal his physical as well as emotional pain and hopefully, his cancer.

First up was the insight that he had never fully committed to life. Entering the physical world had been problematic, to say the least. Stuck in the birth canal, Ronald (and his mother) had almost gone to the grave before he had even been born. The trauma resulted in Ronald's mother longing for the blissful realm of light she had experienced in her NDE, and therefore, committing less to life on the earthly plane.

Such a series of events is a textbook example of a predominantly schizoid/oral character defence. The birth trauma had so intensely influenced Ronald at every stage of his development that he had never fully committed to life, resulting in an underdeveloped first (root) chakra, a tenuous connection to life, and a weakened immune system.

Due to the complications of the birth, Ronald had been unable to breastfeed or receive the necessary nutrition to feel safe and secure. Baby Ronald was bottle-fed by other carers, I guessed, To be bottle-fed by strangers only compensates to a certain degree, because several biological phenomena occur during breastfeeding. The baby has been snugly and safely enveloped inside the mother's womb and her aura during the nine months of pregnancy, and this physical and energetic holding in safety happens again when suckling. Also, the nipples contain a minor chakra, or energy centre, which means in practical terms that the baby not only receives milk but also energy from the mother.

For Ronald, the series of events during his birth proved quite a burden to carry. Such a traumatic event leaves an energetic imprint if it doesn't receive the attention it needs in order to loosen its grip on the individual for them to heal. He had entered the world burdened with guilt about the effect his birth had had on his very arrival, and guilt kept following him. Naturally, the stranglehold of guilt around his mother's near death was completely misplaced, but her son suffered from it, throughout his childhood, into adulthood, and during the final stages of his illness.

As a qualified psychotherapist, Ronald had undergone years of therapy himself and turned the trauma inside out, back to front, and upside down. The therapeutic work on the emotional and mental levels had proved insufficient. The hurtful images had locked themselves away as energetic distortions in his energy body, the aura and chakras, and subsequently his physical body, gnawing away at his insides until they manifested as cancer. In a nutshell, he embodied a classic example of the disease and its origins: a long-term corroding of emotional baggage, an unfolding process accurately befitting the definition of the word *cancer* in Chambers Dictionary (see Chapter 2).

The National Health Service treated him with chemo, according to the oncologist's suggestions. Recovering from the intravenous therapy demanded most of his physical resources. Many of our appointments were spent clearing the energetic debris from the chemo in order to minimize its side effects and for Ronald to maintain a reasonable quality of life. He felt rough, though. His energy levels plummeted, and he looked like a shadow of his former self and found it hard to look in the mirror.

During the remaining sessions we worked on creating further inner clarity, building on the earlier therapeutic work he had done. We managed to clear much of the birth trauma through cleansing and strengthening the relational cord with his mother in both the fourth (heart) chakra, representing the love between parent and child in this case, and the third (solar plexus) chakra, which stores anger, guilt, and shame and governs the digestive system. We cleared guilt over Ronald having abandoned his family when the three children were still very young.

In the ashram ("on the ranch", as he put it), he had acted towards others in ways he only vaguely addressed. We never got to the bottom of certain events. His guilt around these actions seemed too deeply emotionally entangled with shame for him to admit. They surfaced again during our penultimate session, though. The bitterness in his voice was telling, and he was incapable of forgiving himself for his involvement in specific activities, whether participating himself or passively condoning them.

Medically, the situation unfolded in the following way.

Five months after the initial diagnosis, a series of intravenous chemotherapy treatments were completed, and scans showed no cancerous growth but also no significant shrinkage. Ronald had not been shown the scan. He wished to study the first and last scans, and based upon his findings, would decide whether or not to undergo an operation. Around the same time, he received his first injections of mistletoe, a treatment that brought on the anticipated cleansing fevers.

It wasn't until three months later that we met again. He had been on holiday to rest and prepare for the operation, during which almost half of his stomach was removed. With his children living in England, he'd chosen a hospital in their vicinity, but not all of the children were open to visiting him, which unbeknownst to them, fuelled their father's guilt.

Nine weeks of post-operative chemo had been prescribed. During that period we'd scheduled five sessions to clear the energy field and reduce the devastating side effects of chemo, after which we again didn't meet for two months. The latest scan indicated a cancer-free body; however, Ronald experienced severe pains in his stomach and oesophagus when eating and drinking, and weight loss was considerable. "Both your discomforts and weight loss are just a side effect of chemo," explained the oncologist.

Over a period of eight weeks, we met a further five times. It was a time of pure hell for him, during which the medical profession admitted to being puzzled.

About two months before Ronald died we met for the last time. Cancer had been rediscovered and could be targeted by radiotherapy, according to the oncologist, and the following week he would be admitted into a local hospital as a day patient.

On the same day of our last sessions, his wife wrote me the following letter:

Dear Tjitze

First of all a great big thank you for fitting Ronald in today; we both really appreciate it. He was in tears when you offered the session.

I'm writing to you because I am desperate—well, so is Ronald, but he won't beg you, and I will.

I AM begging you—please, please, please, can you find a way to fit in seeing Ronald once a week? I don't know, we don't know, how much longer he has left; his medical prognosis is not good at all. Having said that, we both know that miracles can and do happen, and the one thing that he feels is working (other than the mistletoe, which is more by knowing it would be worse without it) are the sessions with you.

It would not be my normal behaviour to push against your boundaries like this, but I have found that I am doing all sorts of strange things in this process that Ronald and I have been going through. So I am begging anyway.

He wants more than anything (as I think you know) to find peace of mind (well, he would like to live, too, of course) but as he believes you are part of his journey to experience that peace, then I hope you can find a way to see him. If you need to be paid more, then we will find a way to do that.

Regardless of what happens, thank you anyway for what you have already done. Much love and blessings to you.

It was a heart-wrenching letter to read—heart-wrenching to see a man with such wisdom, love, and courage slip away. He had been admitted to hospital a few days later, dragging a worn-out body along, and died there two months later. They were two months of physical hardship and intense suffering. However, when he breathed his final breath he died peacefully, his wife assured me afterwards, much to her and the children's relief. Unfortunately, I was working in Hong Kong temporarily and was also unable to be present when the community celebrated his life.

Guilt had been his life's issue. In the end, it was guilt that consumed his body. In the end, he was not able to fully forgive himself, and a certain amount of self-chastising kept haunting him and prevented health from filtering through into diseased, cancerous cells.

20

Susanne's Story

Type of cancer at our first session: cancer of the blood and in the spleen
Dominant character defence: psychopathic

When preparing to write Susanne's story, I had to check her birth date twice, not believing that she is indeed 50 years old—a young and vibrant-looking 50-year-old woman with unblemished skin and lively eyes. Not that her life has been uneventful. Not in the least, and she has faced her fair share of challenges along the way.

Come to think of it, it is a strange expression: "facing one's fair share of challenges". Fair by whose standards? Who decides what is fair for an individual and what is not fair, enough or too fair? And, when somebody faces no challenges to speak of, is that classed as unfair?

The task of being a single mother of four boys aged between 5 and 15 is no mean feat. She had left a violent marriage the year before she came to see me for the first time, and during the last two years, her health had deteriorated. Pleurisy had led to pneumonia twice and, in turn, had led to septicaemia, resulting in active cancer cells in both blood and spleen.

Blood transfusions and chemotherapy had had the desired effect. The latest tests showed her blood to be normal, controlled by chemotherapy, which she'd been prescribed to take orally for the rest of her life. This was the situation we faced at the time of Susanne's intake.

Behind the bright eyes and strong prescription glasses (due to a slight visual impairment) was a brain filled with visionary thoughts and ideas. It made her speak with passion, vigour, and humour. It soon became clear that she didn't want to live solely to heal her cancer; her aim was to spread awareness among the wider public, that life deserved to be lived to the full. Twists and turns on her road back to health had only served to solidify this vision, which was now even stronger and still growing in conviction.

Our initial session released a big part of memories of violence away from the left shoulder and arm, after which, through guides' spiritual surgery, the blood cleansing and filtering capacity of the liver was rejuvenated during the course of the session. Perceptive as she was, Susanne could feel debris being lifted out of the blood cells.

At the beginning of treatment two, almost four weeks later, she reported that her blood count (see Chapter 11) had not reduced fast enough, according to her oncologist, who had prescribed a 50 percent increase in medication. Her body protested. She started to put on weight immediately, vomited, had spells of diarrhoea, whilst her feet, hands, and arms swelled up.

There was an overall sense of despair in her speech and aura. Why would the body have to go through such an ordeal again? Had it not been put to the test severely enough? Despair overflowed into a sheer now-or-never-kind of desperation, which stimulated her to enter a state of cathartic release of decades of suppressed emotions: fists were flying, feet were kicking, and her voice was shouting in English, Scottish, and slang. The release combined with intricate energetic work freed her feet, hands, and spleen to a large extent.

The release also included leaving behind how Susanne had been programmed and conditioned into the "shoulds" within her family of how her children ought to be raised. Those expectations contradicted her own philosophy of raising and educating them with a sense of freedom of expression, love, and respect. The four children thrived, but standing her ground within the wider family context had been a continuous battle, and still was at times.

Susanne approached her recovery similarly. From her medical team she demanded freedom of expression, love, and respect. From her friends she demanded similar qualities. From herself she demanded nothing less. Thus she embarked upon a voyage of self-discovery with meticulous honesty and precision.

Especially in her attitude towards her family and medical team, Susanne's predominantly psychopathic character defence came to the fore. Someone who displays this type of personality aims to be in control of their life, their surroundings, and any situation that life throws at them. To not be in control feels alien and frightening and needs to be avoided at all costs. Maintaining the vigilance necessary to stay in control takes an enormous amount of energy, but people are rarely aware of their subconsciously held patterns or of the almost continuous draining away of energy. Deep down a person with psychopathic tendencies is incredibly tired but overrides exhaustion through hyperactivity. The way Susanne approached life is an excellent example. She never did anything by halves. Energy spent keeping up a defensive attitude is energy that is unavailable for healing, in Susanne's case, healing her cancer.

She demanded that her oncologist and other medical consultants keep her informed about all aspects of her medical treatment, including medications, procedures, and long- and short-term side effects. She likely raised a few eyebrows along the way, "doing her own thing", not so much disregarding medical advice but distilling every piece of information into her own cocktail of analysis, thoughts, and methods.

All through her treatments she let her body be her guide, paying attention to how it responded to a certain medication, a smaller or bigger dose, to a particular fitness programme at the local gym, and so on. She then mulled these responses in her analytical mind and discussed them with friends and professionals, including myself. Her own analysis and friends' feedback prompted her to grow, both inwardly and outwardly, into a strong, well-informed, and assertive woman.

Her willingness and capacity to absorb information, link it with emotional and physical fluctuations, draw conclusions, and adjust approaches, if and when required, was a joy to follow. Questions were asked by medical doctors, by friends, by me—all of us urging Susanne to deepen her insights, to remain cautious, but not let caution interrupt the tremendously rich flow of life, which surged through heart, brain, nerves, veins, and arteries.

When, for example, her oncologist asked how diligently she took her medication, she replied that she was not always as precise with her intake as prescribed, or words to that effect. A very diplomatic reply, to which the oncologist answered by calling her eccentric in her approach. By that time he had got to know her, appreciate her unusual qualities, and knew how to handle her. She had gained freedom of expression, love, and respect from her medical consultant by being consistent, courageous, and honest. He had learned to appreciate its value.

Not that her journey was always a smooth ride, medically or socially. Her blood count went up and down erratically, an ongoing matter of concern for the oncologist, and at times Susanne couldn't help being affected by his worry. Tuning into her body and what actions it needed from her made her trim her sails according to the wind and be flexible in her approach. Sometimes more rest was needed, sometimes more exercise, sometimes a different ingredient in her diet, sometimes another supplement, sometimes a healing, sometimes a massage. The tactical fluidity served her brilliantly. Rarely does a client exhibit such a consistent in-tune-ness in combination with the soft discipline of inner and outer listening and thus serve her body; most people expect their body to serve them.

Over the years, Susanne faced spells of lower back pain, aching knees, sore feet, flu (a sign of cellular purification), anaemia, strained kidneys, and a yellowing of the skin as her liver worked overtime to detox her body and excrete dead cancer cells and strong medication.

Socially, the simple fact that she was raising four children on her own brought its own challenges, and she often felt stretched to the limit with too little rest, space, and time for herself and for socializing, a typical psychopathic tendency.

At some point, she felt it important for me to get to know all of the boys and sense into the family dynamic and tell her my observations, so we organized a session with all five family members present. First and foremost, it was great fun, for us as well as the kids. It was obvious how much they loved, respected, and treasured their mother without losing anything of their boyish cheekiness and naughtiness or brotherly rivalry.

Susanne benefits hugely from interacting with friends. They support and inspire her to explore new horizons and remain on the right track, so that inner shifts in thinking and feeling keep stimulating recovery on all levels. This stimulation is right up her street. It enhances spiritual opening and strengthens faith in the greater scheme of things, planetary, cosmically, and evolutionarily, never losing sight of how it affects her individual self. In short, Susanne has managed to create a life inside and around her that keeps reminding her to remain the centre of her own life and life's decisions—quite an achievement for a single mother of four children.

A telling example of the way she integrates the different levels of life is how she utilizes the treadmill in the gym. Running physically improves circulation, heart rate, lung capacity, blood pressure, and the immune system through cardiovascular work, and while she runs, Susanne repeats mantras and positive affirmations to the rhythm of her pounding feet. Mantras or positive affirmations can disperse any negative image or belief systems and enhance positive ones.

The pounding footsteps may well serve to get positive statements to settle deeper into her psychological programming, and through that, more solidly into her third, mental, or psychologically orientated chakra, and more solidly into the yellow lines of light of her third, mental, or psychologically orientated auric level. Basically, the treadmill functions to bridge Susanne's mind and body.

This last paragraph sums her up to a T. Creatively, Susanne finds a solution in juggling the limited time she can set aside for herself, and she finds innovative ways to link body, emotion, mind, and spirit.

From the way this chapter has been written, upbeat and light, it will not come as a surprise to you that Susanne is still alive and blossoming. Her story serves as a reminder to not exclude any possibility regarding healing and to include both conventional and complementary approaches. She personifies how beneficial it is to learn to listen to the signals the body sends and act accordingly. She is also a real-life example of how empowering it can feel to take our life into our own hands, even when facing people whom we place in a position of authority, such as (medical) consultants, and how that can ultimately gain us respect even if eyebrows are raised initially.

Try to never lose sight of the fact that healthcare professionals are there to serve their patients or clients, and not the other way around. Susanne utilizes their services for her own benefit and nobody else's. She keeps her empowered attitude to this day.

We still meet occasionally, and mutual respect allows our work together to enter an easy flow of understanding and being understood.

21

Sylvia's Story

Type of cancer at our first session: cancer of the rectum
Dominant character defence: masochistic

It was April 2002. I had just returned from a winter "hibernation" on the Greek island of Skyros and was in the process of settling back in the Findhorn area, temporarily practising from a caravan in The Park, the original campus of the Findhorn Community. Little did I know when Sylvia rang me for a treatment that we were embarking on an incredibly intense cancer journey together over the next few years. She was my first client with cancer, and the first whose complicated healing journey I was able to follow.

Sylvia's presenting complaints at that stage were a long-standing tendency to suffer occasional migraines, chronic poor circulation, numbness of the left foot, and pains in the heart. None of these inconveniences prevented her to live her passion: playing and coaching tennis.

During the intake, it emerged that her first husband had died suddenly in a car accident, 17 years earlier. The deep pain of his loss had been overshadowed by her feelings of betrayal—he had been involved with another woman and had left Sylvia nothing in his will.

We worked intensely on the confusion she felt in her heart, as the combination of grief and betrayal had caused a major tear in her heart chakra. The sudden death of her loved one would have been enough to cause painful feelings of deep loss, but finding out that another woman had usurpesd her place in his heart had done immense damage. Both contradictory and unforeseen happenings had ripped a tear through her heart chakra and disconnected the energy vortex from the energetic line, which connects all chakras, the Vertical Power Current, running from crown to root.

No wonder physical pain surfaced in her heart, migraines tortured her. No wonder there was numbness in her left foot, the foot on the left/feminine/female side of the body: the energetically stored pain prevented her from stepping forward into her innate feminine empowerment (see Chapter 12).

Although she had remarried, during the second session, three months later, it became evident that Sylvia felt trapped in her present marriage, and found her husband so overprotective she felt like she did not have room to breathe or follow her own direction. A key statement was that she blamed herself for not fully committing to him and her second marriage.

Self-blame is one of the characteristics of a predominantly masochistic defence. The person in question always feels that they can do more, try a bit harder, and put a bit more effort into the relationship or into the marriage. At this stage, it didn't cross Sylvia's mind that (at least some of) the fault of their marriage not working to their joint satisfaction might lie with her husband.

Six months later, Sylvia booked a third treatment. This time her presenting complaint was that her guts were playing up. In her words, "I don't have the guts to make the drastic decision to break with my second husband." Without realizing it, Sylvia had uttered a classic masochistic sentence.

The three healings gave her the opportunity to come to terms with grief, rage, guilt, and shame, and physically release those emotions by sobbing, trembling, shaking, and expressing anger. Each session provided new insights, fuelled her inner work, deepened her inner journey, and strengthened her commitment to herself, possibly to the detriment of her marriage.

Still, almost a year later, and two years after our first consultation, the couple was still living in the same house, albeit as estranged partners. The intention of separation had not been fully realized as yet. Symbolic of the situation was that they prepared their own meals and found themselves one evening eating at the same kitchen table at the same time, he with a baked tattie and she with a boiled egg.

Picture the painful scenario for a moment. Two people facing reality by facing each other, with so much more than just a kitchen table separating them. Two people who, in previous years, had shared all that could possibly be shared between two people. A heart-wrenching, gut-wrenching scenario, feeding guilt, shame, and pain, instead of healing it, and seemingly, no way out of their shared misery. A so-called justified escape came in the form of Sylvia being diagnosed with cancer of the rectum.

For many people, the way out of a bad situation comes in the form of a shocking event (the death of a close friend or relative, job loss, dawning realization of previously hidden addiction or abuse, and so forth). The diagnosis of a serious illness can function as a further example. Now, her guts had decided to play up for real. The presenting complaint or symptom or message her body had presented her with almost a year earlier had not received the attention it had demanded of Sylvia.

On the one hand, the time to make a choice of her own free will was past, and her body had made the choice for her by attracting a possibly fatal illness;

on the other, Sylvia was still faced with the need to make choices. Despite, or perhaps because of, her husband clinging onto her, she made a clear decision to heal herself, not him, their relationship, or marriage. She'd made up her mind. She took full responsibility for herself and her well-being and healing. Her husband was no longer her responsibility, nor was the marriage.

What followed was a deeply transformational process for Sylvia. She gradually gained the awareness that she was responsible only for herself and her health, not her husband or marriage, and that healing needed to happen on all levels.

Emotionally, all of the attachment and grudges she felt towards both husbands needed releasing and transforming into love, acceptance, and forgiveness. Mentally, she had to release all of the masochistically stored feelings of guilt and shame she harboured towards both husbands and what she had failed to provide them with, as well as towards both sons. Spiritually, she decided to surrender to God, the Great Spirit, and make peace with her illness, no matter how it turned out—full recovery or death.

Initially, Sylvia took a New Age approach to her healing, allowing only complementary approaches, such as energy healing, counselling, therapy, juicing, detoxing footbaths, and the like, and stubbornly excluding all things medical. Interwoven with this was the inner process of unravelling the marriage, with all its energy-zapping dynamics. Sylvia's husband was clingy, more for the sake of his own pain, fear, and insecurity than for the sake of his wife's healing process. During this time, her youngest son was going through a deeply painful and confusing process in his own relationship on the other side of the planet, in South Africa.

All through Sylvia's healing process, she thus experienced inner battles that took energy away from her need to tackle her cancer. And instead of putting her recovery first, others pulled on her, demanded her time, her attention, her energy—not out of malice or any negative intention towards my client, but simply out of their own neediness and woundedness. Again, notice the masochistic tendencies here of first and foremost looking after her son and husband and putting herself in third and final place.

Very few people are aware of how energetic cords and streamers between individuals work. Interrelational dynamics, consciously as well as unconsciously, determine whether they are sources of energy or deplete an individual of vital resources. When you feel drained after spending time with someone, you may wish to explore how the energy exchange functions and protect yourself if and when another encounter takes place in the future.

In Sylvia's case this tendency climaxed during a visit to South Africa, her home country, a year after her initial diagnosis. At the end of a three-week trip, my notes stated: *Drained during SA: family, wedding, reunion.* Everybody had wanted a piece of her—her time, her presence, her good-naturedness. All of it was understandable, justifiable, fun, entertaining, and . . . exhausting. Above all, exhausting, especially for a woman like Sylvia who had lived a masochistic pattern for decades, centred on pleasing everyone to the detriment of her own wishes, her own freedom of choice, her own health.

In addition, Sylvia found herself trapped between opposing opinions about how to proceed with her cancer and healing, leaving her confused as to which route to take. A friend and medical doctor suggested an operation with a three-month recovery period. Somebody else, with a global reputation in the New Age world and whom she deeply respected, had received inner guidance for her to follow the path of self-healing. A bunch of others had given their perspective and options according to their own beliefs, experiences, or hearsay.

To top it off, on her return to Scotland, several confrontations with her husband took place, partly with and partly without a mediator. All these circumstances turned her cancer, in my visual ESP, into a fiery red and angry blob around the rectum.

Sylvia undertook a series of treatments, including colonic irrigation, a liver and kidney cleanse, spiritual surgery, distancing herself from her husband, widening her horizons, and shedding excess baggage, and as a result the cancer retreated, albeit temporarily.

The feel-good factor took hold for Sylvia, but her hectic social life, together with still playing and coaching tennis, didn't provide her body with enough time and space to recuperate. She lost weight. She started to feel the cold deep in her bones. The first (root) chakra, which energizes the overall immune system, shrank. The lines of light of levels one and three of her aura turned brittle, indicating a weakening connection to the earth, to the physical incarnation (first chakra), and an aura that is losing its ability to feed vital life force into the physical body.

Sylvia's lifestyle became severely constricted within about six months of her tiring trip to South Africa and temporary cancer remission. During these months we cleared emotions and cancerous cells and increased spiritual connections. It was not enough. Something else was required. And that "something else" made Sylvia tumble into a process of surrendering, which she resented strongly.

All of the complementary techniques had proved inadequate, but to admit this naked fact was to admit defeat in her eyes—that she had not done enough, surrendered deeply enough, shown enough faith, cleared enough emotional and mental baggage, and had been unable to connect strongly enough with her spiritual self. The self-chastising displayed exactly the same masochistic pattern as when she had questioned her role during the breakup of her second marriage. In other words, when it came to her health and illness she was not the whole person she aimed to be.

To "go medical" was tantamount to failure in her eyes. In her mind, the choice was black and white: either deliver herself into the hands of the medical profession or continue the inner work in a more disciplined fashion. It hadn't crossed her mind that one approach didn't necessarily need to exclude the other, that a combination of both approaches could be an option.

We spent quite some time discussing the topic, with the result that a fortnight later, she'd paid an initial visit to her GP, had her first test scheduled, and an operation to remove the tumour might follow that next week. In the meantime, she had visited her other son in London and physically crashed in the airport in such an extreme way that she needed medical care, there and then.

During the session afterwards, Sylvia had dreams of fire burning wood. Her lips turned very dry, and she felt continuously dehydrated. She sensed a fire inside and saw visions of "wisps of silvery wind". Gracefully, she kept falling in and out of her body.

These sentences may not make sense to you. Let me explain.

Lucid dreams of fire and dehydration combined with dry lips are signs that the fire element is dissolving, one of the stages a person goes through when dying. According to ancient and well-documented Tibetan wisdom, these are sure signs that death is approaching and physical functions are disintegrating step by step. For more on this, refer to the chapter entitled "The Process of Dying" in Sogyal Rinpoche's book *The Tibetan Book of Living and Dying*, where the dissolving of the fire element is described as follows:

> Our mouth and nose dry up completely. All the warmth of our body begins to seep away, usually from the feet and the hands towards the heart. Perhaps a steamy heat rises up from the crown of our head. Our breath is cold as it passes through our mouth and nose. No longer can we drink or digest anything.

Sylvia's choice to go medical should not have been postponed. Two months later we met again. She had lost a considerable amount of weight and was literally skin over bone. She could only find comfort on the treatment couch on top of layers of extra padding.

The oncologist had suggested a year of chemotherapy, radiotherapy, and surgery, and Sylvia had agreed. The year turned out to be hellish. The broad scale of healings managed to reduce side effects, but she went through agony day after day, night after night. Her 23-year-old son, her youngest, dedicated six months to the care of his mother. His care and that of many other friends, the loving environment of the Findhorn community, and the combination of conventional and complementary methods pulled Sylvia through.

She often left her oncologist stunned, as well as her MacMillan cancer care nurses (MacMillan is a UK based voluntary organisation supporting people with cancer and their families). They were amazed, for example, at how the iron levels in her blood rose unexpectedly, how the tumour shrank after only light doses of radiotherapy, and when finally the operation took place there was not a trace of cancer to be removed.

During the operation the surgeon removed part of the rectum, both ovaries, and the uterus. Afterwards, I saw Sylvia twice in quick succession. That was when, in her own words during her presentation at Findhorn's Love, Magic, Miracles conference years later, I saved her life.

The medical intervention had depleted her already exhausted body, and she was running on empty, with no spare fuel left inside to support her system. She almost had to be carried into my treatment room. On closer inspection, I found that her lower three chakras were disintegrating, as were the lower three levels of her aura. These lower three auric levels and chakras energize the physical, emotional, and mental bodies, the aspects of an individual's life that contain their personality.

At the Barbara Brennan School of Healing, students are instructed to stop all types of treatment when observing this phenomenon, as it will only prolong the dying process and create unnecessary agony for the client. Instead, it is recommended that the practitioner sit with the client in what is termed "the velvet void" to assist the soul in exiting the body and leaving the incarnated personality behind.

How to describe "the velvet void"? More or less, it is perceived as an empty space in between life and death in the physical sense, or an in between space people pass through when in the process of dying physically. It feels soft, open, spacious, dark, and yet not black—dark and simultaneously sparkling.

There is a lightness of being and a warmth that feels ever so welcoming. For a split second a shock wave travelled through me, as the meaning of the disintegration of the lower chakras and auric levels hit me. After all we'd been through and to have this outcome? At that stage in my career I had never before supported a person so intensely through a cancer journey, and to observe Sylvia energetically dying, or preparing for death, seemed totally unjust, undeserved, and deeply painful.

Instantly, my spirit guides took over and demanded: "Restructure, restructure, restructure." I still hear their booming voices, increasing in volume with each repetition of the word. Fortunately, I obeyed the guides and refused to follow our teachers' guidelines.

Needless to say, we made it through this ordeal, Sylvia's final ordeal. Recovery began in earnest afterwards.

Since then, she has remained cancer-free. She plays and coaches tennis again and attends the Wimbledon championship every year, travels the world, walks the Santiago pilgrimage in Spain, is in a new loving relationship, lives a life of service to anyone who asks for her services, serves in the Findhorn Community, and together, she and I support many people in their journey through cancer.

One of the many tools Sylvia used during her journey was to hold a positive vision of the outcome, and in particular, visualizing herself celebrating her 60th birthday in style, with a huge party in Findhorn's Universal Hall.

On her birthday in 2007, weak as she was, her wish came to pass, and Sylvia's Ball filled our hall to the rafters with hundreds of friends. A couple of years later, her son, together with a friend of his, wrote a play with the same name, *Sylvia's Ball,* which they performed in Cape Town, Findhorn, and at the Edinburgh Festival.

She herself performed a single song. For me, it was the first time I'd been made aware of her talents on that front. Never shall I forget how she leaned heavily on the piano to remain upright and sang, accompanied on piano by another community member. Her voice was weak and trembling, but it was her voice, her own voice, singing and celebrating, commencing the next decade of her life.

Sylvia was the first in a long line of clients whom I have supported (or still support) through their illness, and the first to incorporate both complementary and conventional methods in healing her cancer. She was the first to deteriorate rapidly and come back from death's door through our work together, and the first with whom I built a strong professional relationship.

It has etched its relational cords deep into both our hearts. Sylvia had been in the process of dying energetically directly in front of my eyes on my treatment couch when my healing guides stepped in and urged me not to give up. Their booming voices of command and me obeying their prompts resulted in full recovery for Sylvia on all levels.

As an energetic spiritual healer (or whatever you want to call me), I could not have received a more powerful confirmation that one should never give up hope, even in the face of death. My experience with Sylvia increased my faith in our spiritual connections as human beings and in my potential as a healer, and that positivity is something I often share with clients at the outset of a new healing relationship, whether the client has cancer or another malady.

Included in the References is a YouTube clip of a talk Sylvia gave at the Love, Magic, & Miracles conference, organized and hosted by the Findhorn Foundation.

22

One Conversation

Type of cancer at our first session: leukaemia
Dominant character defence: psychopathic/rigid

Richard laughs on entering the treatment room. "Do I look better than last Tuesday?"

It is his style to laugh often, wholeheartedly, and not in the least self-consciously, as if nobody is watching or listening. The laughter and jokes had continued, even when he found himself at death's door in hospital a few months earlier. It is Thursday, two days after the Tuesday he is referring to.

"Yes, you do," I reply. "You look a lot lighter. Did you get plenty of rest?"

"I took it really easy, as you suggested," he says.

"Has life become a challenge now that you're no longer working and you're mainly homebound?" I ask.

"It does bring more tension between my wife and me," he replies.

"I'm not surprised. And how's it for the children?" I ask.

The couple had three boys and a girl. The latter, in her teens, still lived at home. The boys had flown the nest and the oldest had taken over the day-to-day running of the business, which his father had founded some 20 years earlier. He and one of his younger brothers lived together in a nearby town, in close proximity to the business premises.

"They pick up on it. It doesn't overly worry them, though. When my wife discussed it with her therapist, she suggested a session for all family members together to look at our dynamics."

"Family constellation therapy?" I ask, knowing the therapist in question and her speciality. "Excellent idea, and she is good at it. In the meantime, how much energy does this all cost you, and how are you on the whole managing your energies?"

"Pretty good, I would say. Like yesterday, I felt great and wanted to deliver a couple of items to people—things they'd lent me when I was in hospital; a CD player, for example, so I could listen to meditations and lectures. As you know, it supported me greatly.

After I had delivered the first one in The Park [a mile from his home] and had a quick chat with my friends, I needed to drive to Forres [5 miles further], and I didn't fancy the idea. It seemed too long. So I left it for another day."

"Well done for listening to your body and what it needs," I remark.

Richard's choice signifies quite a breakthrough. On earlier occasions, I'd been forced to remind him, often in no uncertain terms, how essential it was to adjust his lifestyle and priorities.

"Do you still feel drawn to the business?" I query.

Richard had created his business from scratch and had made it into a success story, financially as well as ethically. It was his baby. Initially, delegating and reducing his own involvement had been nigh on impossible. Now he is being forced to leave it all to his sons and step back from it altogether.

"No. Of course, I want to hear how it's going, but going back there, no. Last week, my wife had to pick up something, and she asked me if I wanted to come along, and I said no. It's better not to go there."

"Would you run the risk of being sucked in again?" I ask.

"Maybe, but it doesn't feel right to take the risk; therefore, it feels better not to go there at all," he says.

"But not an easy decision, I expect," I observe.

Richard shakes his head. "There's so little I can do, and it annoys me." He falls into a contemplative silence.

"No wonder. As I said before, try to keep seeing this time of non-activity as a time of investment—an investment into a future without cancer; an investment into your health for the next decades of your life."

"I'll never be the same again."

"Possibly. You may never again be able to climb your beloved Swiss mountains. It doesn't mean you'll be unable to enjoy them again at some point in the future, but in a different way. And, you never know. If you give yourself every possible opportunity to recover fully, you can regain your former level of fitness. Just look at Sylvia. She travels the world again, goes to Wimbledon, plays and coaches tennis, the full works. So can you."

"Yeah, she's a good example," he agreed. "I spoke about this with my oldest brother. As brothers, we were often in competition and egged each other on. The last several years, he encouraged me to lose weight, fly over more often, and get fitter by conquering the mountains of our childhood once more, like we've done so often in the past. Now I definitely need to step back from it. And he knows . . . He knows . . ."

Richard bends forward, elbows on knees, and stares into space pensively. "You see, he visited me in hospital just after I had received the severe diagnosis. Before that, doctors gave me an 80–85 percent chance of recovery.

That later diagnosis gave me only a 20–25 percent chance of survival. Up till that point, I'd taken the cancer lightly and thought, *They'll sort me out: you, Thomas, the hospital.* I didn't take it seriously enough."

"That was just when I was in Brazil. Did that make it worse for you?"

"It did. And remember, I emailed you and asked whether you had experience with my type of cancer and you didn't reply a full yes. That shocked me. I saw you as one of the pillars of my support system and probably the most important element in that." The right hand gestures as if holding onto a staff and planting it firmly on the earth in front of him. "Your answer was not what I wanted to hear."

"I can see that, and I'm sorry if that email was a tough one for you at that moment. In hindsight, was it what you needed to hear?"

"In hindsight, yes!" he said. "It threw me back onto myself and convinced me that I had a role to play, the most important role. I had to do something myself and not leave it up to other people, although, I didn't realize that at the time."

"Of course, not. When you're in the midst of things . . ." I agreed.

"You see I was looking for a . . . a . . ." His right hand reaches up, searching for something invisible above his head.

"A lifeline?"

"Yes, a lifeline, and your reply didn't give me that. That was a big blow. And maybe you couldn't."

"I don't remember what I emailed, but it was a difficult situation for us both, with me being on the other side of the planet."

"I understand, and I don't hold it against you. But I was looking straight into the eyes of death, with most likely having to leave everything I loved behind.

My brother arrived the day before that fateful diagnosis. He was present when I received the prognosis. He was shocked. Together, we cried and held hands. He saw me at my worst. And in a way I am grateful for it, because there's no longer any need to explain to him that I will not be able to join him in the mountains. He knows, from having seen me then. It takes the brotherly striving and competition away, which always lingered between us. In a sense that is a relief, a big relief."

Once more he falls silent, pondering. "Why did I have to let it get this far? Why didn't I listen before?"

"That's a key question for many. My guess is that you'll gradually unravel the answer."

"I know the answer. It's guilt. I was only allowed not to work when I wasn't well enough. You will have been brought up in a similar kind of Protestant environment in The Netherlands?"

"With the Protestant work ethic? For sure. Although, religion played no role in our lives. Still, the culture is steeped in it."

"Thought as much. That you can only take time off when you've worked hard for it. Also, only then do you deserve a good income. After hard work."

"You've told me that plenty of times about me and my business."

"Yes, I remember. You deserve a good income and time off because you work hard for it. And, in a nutshell, that's the reason behind my guilt. It's been lingering for years—all my life, really. We grew up with it, and now it is hard to let go of it and relax into doing nothing. The seriousness of the illness now gives me permission to rest, to say no and set boundaries when friends stay too long, for example. Before I would always override my boundaries, thinking I had to be there for them. And then I felt guilty when I asked anybody to leave or when I was too tired to see them. I've been overriding my limits too frequently."

I feel moved. It's just over three months since I returned from working in Brazil. Our sessions resumed as soon as I came back, initially in hospital, then at home, and latterly, with his mobility returning, at my clinic. Despite discussing many related topics, we've never delved so profoundly into his emotional world with regard to my period away, when my client had suddenly been faced with that low percentage of possible survival. Our sessions have focused on the cancer itself, on supporting Richard to make the right choices to enhance his immune system and his strength. Also I feel moved, because the lessons cancer is teaching him are truly starting to take root.

Already this week has proved to be one of celebration. His scan results came back with the most positive news imaginable: no trace of cancer left in the body.

Pretty soon after his last sentence, we start the actual healing session, but this has been a very worthwhile conversation in my opinion, which is why I decided to include it, with Richard's permission. The conversation offers a lesson, I think. I hope it encourages anyone facing cancer to make sure their physical and emotional needs are met at every stage of healing their illness and not be afraid to show their vulnerability in company of their nearest and dearest.

23

Is Cancer Subconscious Suicide?

This chapter was not planned. Nevertheless it cries out to be written. The material came out of the blue as a result of something I am dealing with in my practice, which is teaching me so much. Since it refers to patterns I discuss throughout this book, I feel that not writing it would be a cop-out on my part, demonstrating an unwillingness to confront an uncomfortable truth. Writing, for me, is a way of sorting through events in my life and recording them—fiction or nonfiction, published or not. That is what I have tried to do here.

The events and themes I am about to describe may feel like a repetition of what is written elsewhere; however, for them to come up on four consecutive days indicates to me that together they contain messages, that are too strong to ignore and must be examined.

Last week was a heavy and demanding one and took its toll on me, to the point that when friends paid a surprise visit at about half past five on Friday afternoon, all I could manage as a greeting was a series of long, deep yawns. They understood and didn't hang around.

The focus of that week's taxing workload had been one specific client whom I'd last seen about a year earlier and who had deteriorated severely. She now looked heavily pregnant. Her body was no longer draining bodily fluids of its own accord so they were accumulating around a liver that was swollen way out of proportion. The whites of her eyes had yellowed, as had her complexion.

Eight sessions had been booked—eight sessions of combining psychological and mental inner work with trying to reduce or eliminate the cancer itself, as well as reducing and eliminating pain, for which she had been prescribed morphine, if and when required. A week like that is extremely intense for clients, and their main occupation in between treatments is inactivity or rest. Last Friday she returned to England, pain-free, and with considerable reduction of swelling in the liver area, and her breathing had improved enormously.

A week like that is intense for me as practitioner, too. The involuntary yawning when my friends arrived was a clear indication that my body and mind demanded relaxation.

The diary for this week showed three working days: Monday, Tuesday, and Thursday. Wednesdays are normally set aside for administration, phone calls and the like, and for rest, so it's normally a client-free day. Friday was to be a day of preparation prior to a week of teaching the Bodies of Light course. The three client days were filled with regulars and locals. I did not expect to experience the intensity of the previous week. Some of this week's clients have (had) cancer, some not.

I sighed with relief and told my partner how glad I was that a calm week lay in store. It made her happy, because she can't help but notice the burden this work brings with it sometimes. In the end, though, this was the week that unfolded, another intense one and totally unexpected as such.

Monday

Monday's last client was a man in his seventies, diagnosed three years earlier with lung cancer. Every two or three weeks we meet and keep the situation under control. The only medical involvement is a six-monthly checkup. He'd been a heavy smoker all his life and still puffs his way through over 20 cigarettes a day.

Hip problems mean that he is unstable on his legs, but he managed to go fly fishing frequently last year in the River Findhorn, next to our house. His eyes always light up when we speak about fishing. He doesn't expect to catch salmon any longer, as they may well drag him into the river, but the social aspect of the banter with other fishermen, being outside in nature, feeling the weight of the rod in his hands, casting—the entire scenario gives him a lift.

We are about a month into the new season. Had he been to the river? No. Had he been using the home trainer at home to support his lungs' elasticity? No. He confesses to being too lazy. Instead he arrives about a quarter of an hour before the appointed time, parks the car nearby, smokes a cigarette, then comes in for his lung cancer treatment.

This Monday, I found more energetic mucous on the fourth level of the aura of his right lung than during previous months. I removed it and afterwards informed him of my findings and actions. The man said that coughing had increased and more phlegm had surfaced recently. Energetic and physical symptoms were to be expected. For the umpteenth time, I urged him to move away from smoking in front of the television and increase activity. The choice to remain inactive is a conscious one; so is the choice not to heal; and so is the choice to die of lung cancer after a long and drawn-out illness that leaves you bedridden.

In the English language, there is a perfect aphorism for this man: "You can lead a horse to water, but you can't make it drink."

Tuesday

Tuesday's first client was a local businessman. Whenever business affairs overwhelmed him, the lymph nodes in his armpits swelled up, predominantly on the right. The right side of the body represents the active/male/doing aspects of life; in his case, his business (busyness) life. I can't count the number of times we discussed and analysed cause-and-effect during the last couple of years. To no avail. Busyness and business kept feeding his cancerous symptoms.

About five months ago, he was diagnosed with two different types of lymphatic cancer, a complicated case. He's spent several weeks in hospital, undergone a series of medical interventions, and has found himself balancing on the edge of life and death on a couple of occasions. He's now been discharged and is recovering at home. He's been forced to quit all business involvement—not easy for a man who gave his heart and soul to the success of his business. Nevertheless, he is managing that side of things quite well.

The problem is that it's not enough for him to get up in the morning, have breakfast, read a newspaper, and maybe venture out for a short walk; he needs a purpose. But his body requires him to rest, rest, rest, and rest again if he is to cope with the onslaught of the illness and the after-effects of the various medical treatments.

Herein lies the trap.

When a client's energy levels increase, they may start to feel bored or useless and wish to become active again, but their body isn't ready. How often have I come across this dilemma and pattern in clients.

Five days earlier, he had had a scan, but it was still too early for the results, and he was feeling unduly worried. On another day, he'd felt the need to discuss a sensitive issue with a friend. After that, another friend had popped in and then somebody else. The next day, for the umpteenth time, the lymph nodes in his right armpit were swollen and painful.

The habit of years of overdoing things continued despite his health scare, and the lesson had not been learned. I repeated the sermon he had listened to many a time before. There was fear in his eyes, though, when he asked, "Does this mean that my cancer has returned?"

"Not necessarily," I replied. "But you definitely increase the chances of it returning."

I deliberately choose to speak in the second person at such a moment. It increases the possibility of the message filtering through and encourages the person to change the pattern. The man nodded, understood, and promised improvement. I reiterated that it was a promise to himself, not to me.

I received two phone calls that Tuesday lunchtime. The first was from a client whose story is written elsewhere in this book, who had been to see her oncologist. He'd been unable to say whether her presenting heart flutters and irregularities were a result of chemo's side effects or whether there really was a problem with her heart. To cover all eventualities, he suggested further diagnosis and possible treatments.

The client's question: "Can you please use your High Sense Perception to see if something is amiss with my heart?"

So I entered that still, meditative space, tuned in to my and her guides, and asked for clarification about my perception and messages, and confirmation that they were not wishful thinking on my part but the truth. The truth of my perception was confirmed; namely, that the heart symptoms had been caused by a tightening of heart muscles due to chemotherapy.

Beforehand, the client had consulted another of her therapists, who had also intuitively sensed it to be an irregularity due to chemotherapy. The client was reassured. The first phone call ended.

The second phone call came from the client I had seen for eight sessions the week before. Her oncologist's message on the Monday had been the one every cancer patient dreads to receive: "The only thing we can do for you is keep you comfortable. There's no hope."

To receive the death sentence from a person in authority is devastating. Even more so after undergoing positive treatments at my place, which had removed practically all pain and breathing restrictions. She asked to see me again as soon as possible, convinced that healing still lay within the realm of possibility. The diary had a few gaps a fortnight later. She booked them and said, "My husband will not be happy with it."

Notice those words. This woman had just received her death sentence, so she calls and schedules the only healing option she feels remains to lengthen her life or heal fully, and her first reaction is, "My husband will not be happy with it."

This is the Norwood syndrome (see Chapter 13) in extremis: feeling guilty about her husband even as she tries to stay alive. Is it any wonder my mind sometimes boggles? If she follows her husband's wishes, she will most definitely die within a couple of months, if not sooner. How many women commit suicide like this in order to please their partner, husband, parents, children, and/or friends? How many men, for that matter?

Needless to say, by the end of the Tuesday, I was wrung out, knackered, drained, and frustrated with all these people, who simply don't seem to get it.

As noted, Wednesday is my client-free day. It was a good day. I cycled 40 kilometres, went out for lunch, soaked up abundant sunshine, and felt fit and strong and mellow afterwards. At the end of the day, I tempted fate by mentioning to my partner that the next day, Thursday, was at least going to be easy and straightforward. Well, as it says in self-help books, "Tell God your plans and he'll have good laugh."

At 8 a.m. (9 a.m. in The Netherlands) on Thursday morning, the phone rang. On the line was a Dutch client who I had treated for cancer on and off for over four years. Initially, her medical prognosis had been one year to live, at most, but she took action, went on a fitness regime, and gained the deep respect of all who knew her, inspiring many.

Every year, the annual Tour de France cycling event includes the most gruelling day in the professional cyclists' calendar: the climb up Alp d'Huez. About a decade ago, a Dutch cancer organization started to organize a bike trip, ascending the 21 hairpin bends to to the top of Alp d'Huez, as a way of raising money for charity. The event has grown into an annual red-white-blue-and-orange festival, where the Dutch take over the mountainside for one day.

My client rose to the challenge and completed the climb that next year, and the next. Last year, however, she started the ride against medical advice and had to be taken off the road amidst all these thousands of other cyclists—a huge mental blow for the high-spirited woman. After that blow, her physical situation had deteriorated rapidly, and soon she became wheelchair-bound and unable to travel to Scotland.

She had rung to tell me personally that she had decided to end her suffering and make use of the Dutch option of euthanasia, that she planned to die on Saturday, that she was grateful for the work we had done together. She was very courageous, and her spirit so strong and decisive until the very end. We spoke for about 15 minutes. She knew that eight months earlier my mother had ended her life similarly (see Chapter 15). There and then, the client and I changed our relationship from professional to friendship and shared and cried, each on the other side of the North Sea.

We agreed that she'd let me know the exact time. I'd be teaching a group of ten Bodies of Light students that day, but I promised to interrupt my teaching schedule ten minutes before the exact time of her departure and hold her and her mother and husband in love and light during the transition period. Shattered, I got off the phone.

The second client that Thursday was a local man who was also recovering from cancer. Ten minutes after our appointed time he still hadn't arrived, so I rang to check, as I normally do when somebody fails to turn up. Our appointment had crossed his mind earlier, he explained, but then he had got caught up in a conversation and forgotten all about our meeting. About fifteen minutes later, he arrived, paid, and left and took no time for his treatment. It was, for me, another client's conscious choice to possibly prevent healing, which makes my mind boggle.

Why do people choose not to grab each healing opportunity with both hands in order to heal and prevent cancer from returning? Why do people who are being confronted with such a health scare consciously choose to be so lackadaisical? When they hear stories of somebody else approaching their healing in this way, they may be quick to judge. So why then let themselves off the hook? Cancer will rarely let them off the hook.

Many people who have been diagnosed with cancer make a conscious choice to prolong their suffering or pay the ultimate price of premature death following a long and painful period of being bedridden. As they say, "Many prefer the misery of the known over the mystery of the unknown."

PART III

Cancer and Emotional Imbalances

24

Cancer and Emotional Imbalance

The statement "Cancer is anger internalized", quoted earlier, has been stuck in my brain for years now. Over the years I've questioned its accuracy and relevance. More than two decades of observations have taught me that the statement is too limited. Anger is one of a variety of unpleasant emotions that can be internalized and lead to psychosomatic illness.

In a nutshell: imbalance of the mind (psycho) filters through into the body (soma). Imbalance of the mind can have an emotional aspect (suppressed emotions), a mental aspect (limiting images and belief systems), and a spiritual aspect (lack of faith or a disjointed sense of faith). The imbalance mostly stems from a combination of all three aspects.

If left unexpressed, any emotional imbalance, limiting image or belief system, or distorted sense of faith creates stagnation in the energy field and its two main components: aura and chakras. If such stagnations or energetic blocks remain in place for a short period only, the aura and chakras are capable of cleansing, repairing, and strengthening themselves. It's a normal biological recuperation process geared towards maintaining full health and keeping the species Homo sapiens in existence. The natural energy flow is being restored without the slightest intervention before long-term damage occurs in the shape of some form of psychosomatic illness.

But a long-term energetic block, one that has endured over years or decades, gradually impacts the entire aura and the chakras and their rotating, vital energy, thereby absorbing movement. As a result, restricted chakra rotation allows fewer life-enhancing energies to enter, first, the energetic body, and subsequently, the physical body. This process, in turn, affects the overall immune system (in its entirety or in a specific bodily region, depending on the nature of the suppressed emotion). Finally, the emotion materializes as a physical imbalance; in other words, a psychosomatic symptom, illness, or disease, as we saw with Libby and Evelyn in the introductory chapters.

With emotional imbalances, the emphasis is usually on unpleasant ones that have a negative impact on an individual's well-being, but what about positive ones? Unpleasant emotions have a negative, health-undermining, and immune system–suppressing effect. Pleasant emotions have a positive, illness-reducing and immune system–enhancing effect, because they release endorphins, happy hormones, into the bloodstream. Dr. William Bloom describes this phenomenon in great detail in *The Endorphin Effect.*

The expression "Laughter is the best medicine" rings true because fun is a pleasant emotion and can function as a distraction from a tendency towards mental overdrive and as an immune system booster. YouTube can seemingly perform miracles when you feel down after a devastating medical diagnosis or when you feel exhausted and empty after yet another chemotherapy treatment. Distract yourself for an hour every now and then, not in order to stick your head in the sand and avoid reality but to lift your mood, charge your energy bodies, and boost your immune system. If it makes you laugh, watch Charlie Chaplin, Buster Keaton, Laurel & Hardy, Tommy Cooper, Monty Python, or whoever else might take your humouring fancy.

Hence, when life's challenges seem to get the better of you due to cancer, or illness in general, please remember that your depressed emotional state doesn't need to last. That can also be a choice to a certain degree.

In telling the many client stories in the previous section, I have referred to individual histories and states of being. In the following chapters, I aim to find common denominators and draw conclusions about the correlation between the origin of cancer and emotional, mental, and spiritual imbalances.

25

Complying

Societies have developed sets of norms and values that make living together as individuals within a tribe or society manageable, pleasurable, and fruitful. Such norms and values may not suit us as individuals and may go against the grain of our own priorities, our heart's longing, or our life's purpose. This does not necessarily make the norms and values wrong, nor does it necessarily make our priorities wrong—there may just not be a complete match, or perhaps they don't match for a while, or perhaps they will never match.

What do we do when this occurs? Do we choose our own path regardless of the risk of isolating ourselves socially and becoming separated from the tribe? Or do we comply and sacrifice our own priorities in order to do what is expected as law-abiding citizens?

A similar choice has to be made when two people get together and make a vow (officially or unofficially) to spend the rest of their lives together. It requires compromises and adjustments, naturally, but how far do we allow these compromises to infringe on our individual priorities, our longings of the heart, or our life purpose? Such infringements may subtly creep in, unnoticed initially, or maybe never noticed but considered the normal thing to do in the given situation.

My clients have often provided an illustration of the different ways their life choices have come to impact their lives, attracting cancer.

Take, for example, Archie, who without so much as a grumble, accepted his parents' order to serve as a surrogate father to his younger brother. He subsequently threw himself into a career that allowed him to become a high earner and lived an excessive life style. He did what was expected of him and complied with other people's demands, but overriding his own desires gradually caught up with him. Another turning point came when his father fell ill some 18 months prior to Archie's cancer diagnosis. Again, Archie fitted in with his father's requests or demands and did as he was told.

Or Josh. The dynamics between her and her husband had been a prime cause of her holding back her essence, clipping her wings and freedom of spirit and leading to self-criticism, and her sweetness had become her downfall. Digging into her childhood had revealed situations where rage seemed utterly justified, but suppressing those emotions had been an easy way of keeping the peace. Josh took it upon herself to be the guardian of her younger sister, and her own grief was swallowed in the process.

Richard had told me that, growing up, he had been allowed to take time off work only when he was unwell. He suggested that the Protestant environment and work ethic was to blame, making it hard to take time off unless you have worked hard enough to have earned it and only then deserve a good income as a result.

Patricia was the sunshine child in her family and smiled her way through her childhood. She had never complained, agreed with virtually everything, looked after her younger sister, and performed all manner of chores without prompting. She wanted to please her mum, but in such a way, that she would pay less attention to her, not more, because Patricia's mother didn't give her daughter the space she longed for. What she longed for more than anything else was for her mother to be genuinely interested in her. Among her friends, too, Patricia had been known as a merry lassie, or at least a girl who outwardly tried to portray a merry lassie, giving generously despite feeling lonely deep inside.

Pauline also had supported her mother devotedly, but fear had been holding her back all of her life, especially fear of her stepfather. He dominated, manipulated, and often turned to violence, physically and sexually targeting both females.

In Susanne's case, in order to liberate and empower herself she had to unlearn the patterns she had been programmed into, including the family expectations of how her children ought to be raised.

Sylvia, too, had to learn to take responsibility for her own life and health, not for her husband and their marriage despite her husband clinging onto her, more for the sake of his own pain and insecurity than his wife's healing process. Besides that, everybody wanted a piece of her—her time, her presence, her good nature, because that's what Sylvia's near and dear ones had grown used to through her pattern of putting others in first place.

~

Dynamics such as those I highlight above, and in the clients' stories in the previous section, gradually create unsettledness in the person involved. They, almost as a norm, feel torn between following their own instincts and needs on the one hand and on the other hand the wish to please and pacify others. This is an excellent feeding ground for inner battlefields.

The weighing up of pros and cons seems pretty harmless on the surface. It is, initially. As years go by, though, the suppressed inner longing reveals itself to be just that: suppressed, placed on the back burner, for it to be moved to the foreground at a later stage or never addressed.

A couple, for example, may reach the agreement for the man to remain the breadwinner and focus on his career and prospects while the woman focuses on raising their children, a decision in alignment with society's traditional norms and values and, therefore, not in the least disagreeable. The woman complies, and a new status quo has been achieved effortlessly—at least on the surface. But below the surface, unnoticed, an inner conflict or dissatisfaction may well arise as an ever-increasing corroding force. The process can contribute to the onset of a variety of psychosomatic illnesses, including the possible awakening and stimulation of cancerous cells, by undermining inner equilibrium with all its side effects in the aura, chakras, and immune system.

We saw this with Patricia. A red blob appeared in her aura around the liver, the organ that stores anger and rage. As a result, the aura around her pelvic region became more activated, as if something was brewing beneath the surface. During one specific session, it became the most significant auric feature, and red was the dominant colour in her energetic field.

In psychology, this type of emotional regulation is called Expressive Suppression. The phenomenon is typical of people who do not show their true emotions. It is a conditioned behavioural pattern born out of the experience that expressing the full emotion might worsen a situation, increase conflict, deepen an argument, and increase the risk of abandonment, violence, or other unpleasant dynamics. A person in such a situation easily remains quiet and withdrawn in order to avoid the limelight.

When somebody chooses to remain invisible the aura automatically contracts and becomes denser, reducing energetic circulation and distribution into and throughout the physical body. The impact is instant. Its effect can be measured as a reduction of the person's energetic frequency in body and aura. Compare this to the immediate shift in measurements of the pendulum swing when one student read a classmate's crown chakra (Chapter 43).

When science begins to pay more attention to the correlation between physical and energetic surroundings, huge progress can be made in the development of healthcare and prevention of illness. Serbian-American inventor Nikola Tesla, who did extensive experiments with electricity observed, "The day science begins to study nonphysical phenomena, it will make more progress in one decade than in all the previous centuries of its existence."

26

Grief and Sadness

Grief is an emotional state that most of us wish to leave behind as soon as possible. When a close relative or friend has passed, or a certain event has happened, triggering an association with loss, such as divorce, redundancy, moving home, it can "pull on the heart strings".

The expression has significance in the most literal sense of the word. Heart strings exist energetically. We call them "relational cords" (see Chapter 8). We develop relational cords from each of the seven main chakras with anyone we relate to, whether through family ties, a friend, acquaintance, neighbour, or colleague, even a brief meeting on a bus, train, or plane.

Relational cords establish themselves between our heart centres, or heart chakras (not to be confused with the physical heart), as soon as love, affection, passion, or compassion are involved, whether mutual or one-sided. When a relationship changes, the energetic flow along the relational cord also changes.

It means that when contact is lost, abruptly or gradually, our emotions are affected. Most of us feel that we are no longer able to share the particular quality of love associated with the deceased or departed significant other. That simply hurts. In order to avoid the intensity of the emotion, we tend to avoid thinking or speaking about the lost one and bury the pain.

In energetic terms, it impacts the relational cord with the loved one, rooted in the fourth (heart) chakra. The cord no longer tips directly in the chakra's centre (avoidance) or becomes thinner, brittle (less or no energy is being exchanged and/or the energetic flow becomes one-sided) or will be torn (depletion of the heart's capacity to love, often resulting in a closing down of the heart due to painful separation).

Our lungs are situated directly on either side of the heart chakra. They can bear the brunt of the heart's energetic depletion through grief, because the heart is the energetic centre that absorbs universal life force for both lungs.

In the case of my client Adam, who had lost his wife, I made a few initial attempts to support him in entering a grieving process to try and release the dark cloud of stagnated energy that had his heart, lungs, and chest in a vice-like grip, but the man avoided direct questions by falling silent, just staring into space. On several occasions Adam made it clear that with some kind of evasive remark he wanted me to stop questioning him about the loss of his wife.

If you'll recall, Sylvia's husband had died suddenly in a car accident. Her deep loss had been overshadowed by feelings of betrayal when she found out that he had been involved with another woman and as a result had left her nothing in his will. The combination of grief and betrayal ripped her heart chakra apart. No wonder physical pain surfaced in her heart centre.

When she was diagnosed with cancer three decades later, it was located in her rectum not in an area close to her heart centre. Grief and betrayal of the heart had not been the only traumatic dynamics during the intervening years, although they may well have undermined her immune system to such an extent that she was unable to cope with an added emotional onslaught.

The truth was, Sylvia felt trapped in her second marriage and found her husband's attentiveness and overprotectiveness stifling. A key sentence was that she blamed herself for not fully committing to him and their marriage. Had she failed once more? After the painful events around her first husband, the feelings of restriction became too much to swallow, too much to digest, too much to rid herself of internally. The result? Her digestive tract and, specifically, her rectum, had been affected.

When traumas of a different character are being added during various stages in life, minor health scares can occur. They can be dealt with accordingly, but at some point, the body fails to cope with the totality of trauma and a serious illness starts to take hold. More often than not, the digestive system takes the brunt. When we pile our plate full of food and eat the lot, including starter and dessert, it is our digestion that protests. When we store trauma after trauma in our body, protests can easily stem from our digestion.

Ronald's story is also a prime example of this phenomenon. His plate overflowed with difficult-to-stomach emotional baggage, which was perhaps impossible with his heavy-handed and guilt-laden approach to life. At some point a year and a half before I treated him, the man had been hospitalized with stomach trouble and an endoscopy had revealed active cancer cells. Later on during his disease process, a scan showed a thickening of the stomach lining and an affected duodenum.

In Julia's case, her father had passed away when she was young, and she hadn't been allowed to attend the funeral. As a result, sorrow and guilt were embedded in her grieving heart. Cancer had been diagnosed in her breast, pectoral, and intercostal muscles, all situated around the heart in the physical area energized by the heart chakra.

Is it a coincidence that there is a correlation between the physical location of the energy centre (heart chakra) and the disease location? Of course, but is it truly coincidental? The sheer number of examples of client background stories and presenting physical illnesses would seem to be proof that there is correlation that can neither be overlooked nor ignored.

Similarly, when a person finds it too challenging or painful to come to terms with a series of traumatic experiences over the years, isn't it common sense to assume that an overload can turn out to be either too hard to "swallow" or "stomach", as the sayings go in English? Is it any wonder the digestive tract (from oesophagus to rectum) starts to show psychosomatic symptoms after a while?

As an exercise, if you know somebody with cancer of the digestive tract, I invite you to take a moment to reflect on what life events they may have been unable to digest emotionally over the years or decades. Now do the same for somebody with cancer in other parts of the body, and try to figure out what emotions that body part may have stored over the years. See if you can find a correlation between the affected physical area and the person's life.

Of course, you should not expect to know the entire emotional baggage of a person. As we've seen earlier, when someone complies with society's norms and values, many physical, emotional, mental, and spiritual issues can remain well hidden from the outside world. Sometimes though, a link may be obvious. Now do the same for yourself. It's equally difficult.

You'll never know the full background and impact of someone else's past issues, not even your own. Idealized self-images need to be put aside, along with some ego, and links between past and present may need to be reflected back to you by somebody else, be they friend, family member, acquaintance, or professional. By no means is this an easy process, but it is worthwhile because it offers a chance to make an investment in a future with a strengthened sense of inner peace.

27

Worry and Frustration

The words "worry" and "frustration" both depict a state of mind that is unsettling to say the least, but in my view they are inextricably linked. When a person is frustrated because something isn't moving forward fast enough, seems too complicated, or may take too much effort, more often than not worries take the upper hand. The mind creates an ongoing train of thoughts running riot in the brain like a hamster on a wheel, going round and round without actually getting anywhere.

The subject of the train of thoughts is irrelevant and can range from how to improve intimacy within an existing relationship to whether there'll be enough time to make a connecting flight at the airport. Whatever the subject, the mental overdrive takes the person out of the present, projects into the future, and creates what are usually worst-case scenarios.

How is this relevant to disease and the healing process? Simply that an over-burdened mind weakens the mental chakra, or third (solar plexus) chakra, and the yellow lines of light of the mental auric level, the third level (see Chapter 3).

When a client speaks negatively about the possibility of healing, their life's circumstances as a result of a cancer diagnosis, side effects of chemotherapy, and so on, they are often completely unaware of their negativity. Certainly, rarely is a person aware of the negative impact of their negativity on both aura and chakras.

When I hear a series of negative statements, I repeat some of those sentences back to the client and explain the energetic differences between positive and negative phrases and how they influence their energy body in opposite ways. My role as a healer is not just about performing healing techniques but about the client leaving the treatment room with better self-awareness and a new set of tools to facilitate self-healing, along with a renewed self-responsibility and a stronger sense of self-empowerment.

Frustration was my client Luciana's main issue—frustration about the slow recovery process; frustration about the risk of the illness rearing its head for a fourth time and the ever-present need to remain vigilant; and frustration about not working and not contributing to society and the joint marital income. She felt a continuous level of frustration, resistance and general pissed-off-ness over what life threw at her. Rarely was she upbeat, lighthearted, or blessed with a trouble-free mind when she entered my treatment room, despite being a "walking miracle".

In Chapter 23, a local businessman struggled after he was forced to retire due to his health problems and give over the running of his business to his son. Getting up in the morning, having breakfast, and having nothing to do but read the newspaper and maybe venture out for a short walk was unsatisfying to him. He needed a purpose.

When he turned his attention to work, though, albeit only in his ever-analytical mind and not in any practical manner, the lymph nodes in his armpits swelled up again on the right side (the right side of people's bodies represent the active/male/doing aspect of life). The man's body gave him clear messages that worries and an overdose of activity of the mind affected his physical health negatively each time he tried to return to work.

This client is typical of someone who has (had) cancer, is beginning to recover, and whose energy levels are increasing. When that's our sense, we easily and often quickly conclude that we can return to some sense of normality. What the person in recovery forgets, or is unaware of, is that it can take much longer for the physical body to fully regain health. Our physique is the densest part of our being, so it takes the longest to catch up after a disease process and medical intervention. The mind might feel confident and physical limitations feel highly frustrating, to the point that a person often feels tempted to override these limitations. If a person becomes active too soon, though, the already battered and bruised immune system is unable to keep up, and cancer may well return in the same physical area, or elsewhere.

In Josh's case, she did not want to die and leave her daughter, the apple of her eye, to be raised by her husband, who she felt had neither the sense of responsibility nor the maturity to raise the child on his own.

Julia, meanwhile, felt pressurized to apply for a job when her husband lost his, and part of her resented having to sacrifice a chunk of her precious time that she wished to dedicate to her healing journey.

All three of these clients are examples of how ongoing worry and concern unsettle a person's mind and inner peace. In such a situation, how often does the mind wander, wonder, and question whether the desired solution will be achievable, and if so, when, where, with whom, and why not already? Every time thoughts drift in the direction of worry or concern, energy drains away from the present into a future state of being, into a longing to reach a desired goal, achievable or unachievable. By not living fully and whole-heartedly in the present, the aura contracts, becomes more dense, and one or more chakras become dysfunctional. In this case, the first (root) chakra literally uproots the person from the here-and-now—a here-and-now that leaves much to be desired. A disconnection takes place. The energetic uprooting. This can either mean that the rotating funnel of the individual's root chakra doesn't reach deep into the earth or doesn't reach deep enough into the person's physical body.

When the chakra doesn't reach deep enough into our planet, the stabilizing, nurturing, and nourishing vitality of the earth is not fully tapped; and when the chakra doesn't reach deep enough into a person's physical body to make a functional connection with the VPC, it may receive power from the earth but be unable to distribute it where aura and physical body need it.

My client Patricia's root chakra seemed not as deeply sunk into the earth as ought to be expected, and the tip of the chakra seemed not fully connected to the energetic anatomy of her overall system. My ESP indicated that there was a clear disconnection between Patricia the individual as incarnated being and the earth upon which she was incarnated. This energetic and physical tendency is part of my client's schizoid defence structure, resulting in an underdeveloped root chakra, which, in turn, can lead to an underdeveloped immune system, because it is our root chakra that energizes our immune system.

Either way, the body is unable to absorb the full quantum of earth energy. As a result, the lower pelvis and its (reproductive) organs will become depleted, including the testicles, ovaries, and bladder, and the kidneys and adrenal glands can be undernourished. Although not physically in the same region, these organs are being energized by the first chakra.

To complete the picture, if that same person lives in an almost constant state of worry of attracting a serious illness, cancer included, they increase their chances of attracting exactly what they fear most by entering and remaining in a state of fear, thereby compromising their root chakra and immune system in what becomes a self-fulfilling prophecy.

That's what happened with Luciana. From an early age she'd had an unexplainable fear of dying young and of falling victim to a serious illness and felt that these beliefs prevented her from achieving her aim of returning to full health.

Worry and frustration create the desire to live elsewhere, with somebody else, with a different job, and to swap the present for an idealized future; in other words, worry and frustration can cause an internalized wish for moving, uprooting. The inner and/or outer process of uprooting, or the secret, unexpressed wish to do so, affect the root chakra negatively and can lead to malfunctioning kidneys and adrenal glands and the overall immune system.

28

Fear

The emotional charge of fear is a huge one. It is the emotion I come across more than any other in my work with cancer clients.

The first instinctive physical reaction to fear is for people to hold their breath. The first energetic reaction is a reduction in the charge of the first chakra, because of experiencing a physical threat. Simultaneously the entire aura contracts and becomes denser. Both result in a sudden reduction of energetic flow and circulation.

When sitting opposite a client during our chat prior to an actual healing, I notice these physical and energetic reactions time and time again. Most of the time, I make clients aware of my observations, not in order to tell them off or humiliate them but in order for the client themself to gain more self-awareness.

Also, as I've stated on several occasions, fear creates the tendency in people to try and escape from reality, to try and escape from the here-and-now. As soon as the first flicker of a wish to escape crosses our mind, without realizing, the first chakra instantly reduces its connection to the here-and-now, to planet Earth. We "pull up the drawbridge", the root chakra, which governs kidneys and adrenal glands. That is why these organs are associated with and affected by fear. Long-term exposure to fearful situations may be detrimental to the functioning of those organs.

Adrenal fatigue, for example, is nothing but a physicalized fearful state of being. It often relates to an indirect fear, one that doesn't necessarily threaten the person's life directly but is more an underlying fear arising from abuse, violence, poverty, abandonment, and other factors that lasts years or decades. It is based upon previous experiences and is subconsciously tucked away somewhere in the body for it to fester.

Besides absorbing the vital life energy of these areas of the body and organs, the root chakra is responsible for keeping an individual's overall immune system in good health.

It's important to realize the implications. If a person lives in a prolonged state of fear and wishes to be elsewhere, his overall capacity to live is reduced, possibly to the point of annihilation. Interesting or what?

As I pointed out, it's as if the person pulls up the drawbridge energetically and the root chakra reduces in size and vitality. Knowing that that same first chakra regulates the overall immune system, it becomes of paramount importance to reduce fear as much as possible during a client's daily life.

In this respect it is very unhelpful (to use an understatement) for the medical profession to present a patient with a worst-case scenario when informing them of a diagnosis and a prognosis.

In Luciana's case, I noticed that she was bombarded by fear and devastation and rarely managed to relax her ever-active mind. Her mental tension showed strongly in the third mental level of her aura.

And Ronald had little faith in life, especially his own, which he considered undeserved. This contracts a person's aura and chakra system as well as DNA strands and leaves them wide open to all manner of daily negative influences. The impact of these is even stronger when the energetic buffer zone (the aura) has lost much of its fluid expansiveness, its coping mechanism.

This type of impact is not conducive to anybody's health. Whether an aura functions optimally or not can make the difference between one person contracting a serious illness and another person avoiding it. Someone with a (serious) disease or who is recovering from one can ill (pardon the pun) afford energetic depletion. Physical as well as energetic bodies need every ounce of energy available to them during the stages of illness and recovery.

Another source of fear is that of dying young, before a full and fulfilling life has been lived, and/or that of attracting some life threatening illness, another feature of Luciana's case. What kind of a role did this young woman's belief system play in her attracting cancer?

Pauline had a similar fear. Her mother had suffered for two years with progressive ovarian cancer and had been bedridden before death put an end to two years of agony. Pauline had nursed her mother through this period and had been strongly affected by watching her mother grow weaker. The gruesome images kept haunting her daughter, and she began to develop the belief system that she was also fated to succumb to the same illness. Sure enough, a couple of decades later she developed ovarian cancer.

Had Pauline grieved sufficiently? Had she managed to put her mother and her two-year-long dying process at rest, devastatingly painful as it had been to witness for the devoted daughter? During these years, to what degree had Pauline overidentified with her mother? To what degree had she intended to carry some, if not all, of her mother's burdens, pain, suffering, or even some of the cancer itself to try and relieve her of some of her agony?

Most likely, Pauline's overidentification with her mother's fate had been instrumental in creating her debilitating belief system, which had fed cancerous cells energetically in a self-fulfilling prophecy. Her mindset of doom-and-gloom reduced the energetic flow in both aura and chakras and created a feeding ground for cancerous cells to multiply and spread.

When working with a client whose thought patterns follow a similar pattern to Pauline's, I basically follow two approaches.

First, I try to disentangle the mother's relational cords in the client's chakras. I do not cut or remove them, but instead, cleanse them, repair them, and try to achieve a healthy two-way flow between mother and daughter. By doing this, the debilitating overidentification can be reduced or halted completely and the client grows more strongly into her own identity, independent from the other.

In Patricia's case, I worked with her relational cords during our third session. The third (solar plexus) chakra opened wider and deeper than before, and lots of sadness and anger came out of her throat and jaw, and she screamed and pounded her fists on the couch in unbridled rage.

This is an essential step for all individuals at all times: shifting from dependency to independence, or a healthy mutual interdependence, based upon an equal flow of two-way communication.

Second, I verbally emphasize that mother and client are two very different individual human beings—intricately related, yes, but each with a unique past, present, and future and each with a very different life purpose for this incarnation.

So in Pauline's case, I said:

> You are not your mother, Pauline. Your mother was not you. You each have very different lives to live. Both you and your mother were born under very different circumstances. Both you and your mother will live and die under very different circumstances. That's okay, because that's how it's meant to be for two different individuals, whether they're related or not.

It may well be that I repeat some of these phrases later on in the session and/or during next sessions. Repetition can serve to keep bringing the message home and verbally support the effect of the disentanglement of relational cords.

Yet another source of fear is that instilled by society, where cancer is portrayed as the big killer, the big enemy, more dangerous than any environmental impact or terrorist organization. The danger lurks in all nooks and crannies.

On one occasion, Patricia became scared when directly adjacent to where the needle of a hormone injection had penetrated her skin she discovered a painful lump. This was by far the most alarmed I had seen my client and resulted from a standard medical procedure.

Attracting cancer is an invisible risk, and whether somebody gets cancer or not can be nothing more than a matter of luck or bad luck—this was the conclusion drawn by researchers from Johns Hopkins School of Medicine in a 2015 study that received a lot of media attention. As reported in a 13 January 2015 article by Ruth Alexander in *BBC News Magazine* entitled "So, Is Cancer Mostly 'Bad Luck' or Not?" (https://www.bbc.com/news/magazine-30786970), ... "the researchers say that they have calculated that two-thirds (65 percent) of 'the differences in cancer risk among different tissues' is down to cell division gone wrong: 'bad luck'. Now many media reports have simply concluded that this means that two-thirds of cancer cases are just the result of random haywire cell division. That's not correct. But on the other hand, a lot of people aren't quite sure exactly what the researchers mean."

Well, that's misleading journalism. The shortest sentence in this quote is the most important one: "That's not correct." Most people will not read it but restrict themselves to reading and remembering the headlines. Almost every TV, radio, and newspaper report that day carried a variation of the headline "Cancer is Just Bad Luck."

Do people believe in luck? Most do not. They expect the winning lottery numbers to drop into somebody else's hands, a luckier person than them, and pass them by. However, people do believe in bad luck.

To me, the above article is an extreme example of how local, national, and international media portray cancer—strongly fear-based. The general public can easily be taken in by media reports and fall into the trap of feeling unable to influence their own health after registering such headlines. Frequently, people lean towards an attitude of apathy in relation to cancer prevention and cure. They feel at the mercy of those in power, that is, medical and state authorities, and accept their diagnosis, prognosis, and future treatment plan as gospel.

This type of journalism promotes apathy and increases fear. It also creates or bolsters the incorrect belief that individual actions in preventing cancer are futile. Susanne is an example of someone who learnt how empowering it can feel to take life into your own hands, even when facing authority figures such as medical consultants, engendering respect even if the initial reaction is raised eyebrows.

The medical profession is responsible for instilling a lot of fear in patients with cancer. When you are the one receiving the report, diagnosis, and prognosis, no longer is the professional speaking about somebody else, in some faraway country, distant county or city, the next street, or neighbouring house; instead, it concerns the person living underneath your own roof, the person sleeping in your own bed, the person living inside your own skin: you. It is often a shocking revelation.

In Luciana's case, during the course of our work together, on one occasion a consultation with her oncologist undermined our progress temporarily and instilled a great deal of fear in her. The oncologist had been cautious regarding the scan results, and his caution undermined Luciana's already fragile sense of trust and made fear flare up. As a result, she had visibly contracted energetically. After that, every time she was due for a scan she became nervous, and whenever the results were due she was scared.

Josh's life expectancy was just six months when she consulted me initially. Her diagnosis of cancer of the liver six months earlier had come as a great shock. Her biggest fear was death. Not really for her own sake, but, as alluded to earlier, for her daughter's.

Susanne's blood count went up and down, a matter of concern for the oncologist, and at times Susanne couldn't help but be affected by his worry.

In chapter 22, Richard states: "Before that they gave me an 80–85 percent chance of recovery. That diagnosis gave me only a 20–25 percent chance of survival. Up to that point I'd taken cancer lightly. But I looked death in the eye directly, with most likely having to leave everything I loved behind."

And one last extreme example offers still further proof of the impact of fear on the body. The woman whose picture I painted inside "Julia's Story" was threatened and robbed and died days afterwards due to ". . . an abnormally aggressive spread of cancerous cells all over her body".

How can science explain this, other than it being an existential trauma causing her entire body to be riddled with aggressively active cancer cells within days? Proof, especially after an official medical autopsy, that disturbed emotions and cancer are strongly related.

29

Guilt and Shame

In this chapter I cover guilt and shame. I've placed these emotional issues under a single heading because they are intrinsically related and energetically interwoven. The third (solar plexus) chakra is concerned with the position we occupy in society. If we feel that we have failed to attain the powerful, influential position we expected to occupy in life, shame and guilt may play a role in our life.

That "position" is different for different people. It may involve financial security for our retirement years or perhaps job security and income in order to provide for our family. These, in turn, depend on where we are on our career ladder, the type of study, qualifications, and educational institution we graduate from, or even the secondary or primary school we attended as children. This social pressure knows no gender. It affects us all.

Notice that I said "expected to occupy" in that first paragraph, implying that there's somebody who expects a certain attitude, behaviour, career, and achievement from us. Who is the person expecting and thereby putting pressure on us? Is it self-imposed, or is the pressure coming from society in general? The key here is who expects what from us and how far we internalize such expectations and make them falsely our own—a link to the previous chapter on "complying". How far do we comply with what is expected of us and thereby lose sight of our own ideals and preferences?

Initially, during childhood, the person who expects something is the parent, or both parents, who put pressure on the child to reach a certain standard of attainment, mainly in their school reports, but possibly in sporting events, creativity, and the like. Later, teachers demand results and when the child fails to meet these expectations, guilt and shame kick in. This can have a strong effect on self-esteem, leading to self-blame, self-chastising, and self-hatred (see Chapter 25).

At this point, childhood conditioning is complete, and a pattern of avoiding failure in the eyes of the spouse, offspring, friends, neighbours, boss, manager, or colleagues has been set in motion that leads us to override our own desires and comply with other's needs to avoid being put on the spot, shamed, and singled out.

Maintaining this behaviour takes tremendous effort, but because it has become the norm, the exhaustion associated with it goes unnoticed.

Guilt and shame are connected with how we relate to our social surroundings, to the people around us, and are thus most easily visible in the way the relational cords in our third (solar plexus) chakra are functioning. Many of these cords will end in our third chakra with a hook at the end, indicating that we are literally hooked by the expectations of others in our social circle, limiting our individual freedom. When the issue involves a repetitive pattern, a few or many of these cords become entangled or even tightly braided together. Those cords need disentangling for healing of that particular recurring pattern.

What I've witnessed on many occasions is that the disentangling and dissolving of the cords happens spontaneously when my client has fully grasped the why, what, and how of the recurring pattern. Once they manage to integrate a different attitude and relate in an empowered fashion to the demands of people around them (who, most likely, will not have realized the impact of their demands), the cords lose their negative charge. They become smooth and light, and energy flows in both directions in equal measure.

Feelings of guilt and shame undermine the functioning of the third (mental, solar plexus) chakra. This chakra's psychological significance has to do with the sense of self within society, including the relationship with social surroundings of family, friends, colleagues, and so on. Guilt and shame disrupt a person's natural inclination to relate from a sense of inner peace, security, and contentment. These dynamics cause the third chakra to become distorted. In turn, the chakra fails to function optimally and rotate healthily; hence it fails to absorb the vital life energies necessary for the physical functioning of the digestive system, governed by the solar plexus.

Ronald, for example, had entered the world burdened with guilt, and it kept following him. Any sense that he deserved pleasure had been eradicated, to the point that it even turned his joy in writing into an exercise in self-chastisement. He looked physically burdened, and burdened himself still further with his single-minded approach to everything. In his mind, he had reasons aplenty to justify feelings of guilt—he had been stuck in the birth canal prior to being born and his mother had almost died. Ronald had deserted his family in England in order to join a renowned ashram in India, and his children had difficulty forgiving their father for abandoning them. In the ashram, too, Ronald undertook actions towards the public that he only vaguely addressed, but he felt such guilt and shame about these actions, he could not admit to them. Guilt and shame had brought on stomach cancer, and when Ronald was dying in hospital after his final operation for cancer, not all of his children were open to visiting him, which only fuelled their father's feelings of guilt. Guilt had been his life's issue, and in the end it was guilt that consumed his body. Guilt and shame, and Ronald's inability to come to terms with the complexity of the issue, cost him his life in the end.

Guilt also played a big part in Julia's inability to heal her breast cancer. In her case, it was strongly tied up with a search for love, for fulfilment of the heart, and feeling torn between two men. It quickly became apparent that her heart was torn, and the relational cords were entangled, as feelings of loyalty towards her husband battled with a rekindling of love and romance with her lover. The inner battle ripped her heart apart. Although she responded very positively to our first series of treatments, the inner turmoil of guilt around her love affair played havoc with her battered, bruised, and seriously challenged immune system. Ultimately, it undermined any chance of recovery.

Guilt and shame are triggered when we relate to others from a distorted sense of self or other. "Other" in this case refers to a group of people: family, colleagues, team-mates, and the like. When someone's sense of self or other has been distorted through conditioning or programming, they feel unable to act, speak, or live authentically when they are with others. A sense of spontaneous enthusiasm is lacking. They lack a positive sense of self within society, and the third chakra suffers, as does the physical region that it is supposed to energize: the digestive system.

30

Anger

Without a sense of humour, the intensity of work with people on the edge of life and death can quickly become too heavy a burden to shoulder. I'm laughing at myself here, because we're in the final phase of assembling this manuscript and I suddenly realized that I've totally forgotten to include a chapter about anger.

One of the phrases I like to use when teaching students about anger is that it is an emotion that is avoided more frequently than any other. So what do I do myself during the process of writing this book? I simply "forget" the topic of anger due to my own subconscious avoidance, perhaps.

The expression of anger often results in an outburst of violence—physical or verbal, but most definitely energetic—and perhaps that is one reason we avoid it. If the angry person is alone and experiences an outburst without anybody at the receiving end, there's no direct damage done. But if someone is in the vicinity, they may feel threatened and frightened as a result, even when the anger is not specifically directed at them.

Do not underestimate the energetic force of anger. Energy moves with the speed of light and bridges distances effortlessly. Angry energies, thoughts, or intentions reach the person to whom they are directed in a flash, whether the source of anger and the recipient are in close proximity to each other or not. So as a word of caution, try to be aware of how you use your emotional charge, especially anger. Avoid directing any outburst of anger in someone's direction, It will not serve you and may cause damage, fear, and mistrust in the energy bodies and/or in the mind of the receiver.

The expression of anger is a powerful force, a force to be reckoned with; however, avoiding and suppressing it is equally damaging, as it gets dammed up and stored in the body for years, decades, and those forceful energies gather and await eruption. The organ associated with anger is the liver.

My HSP often tells me whether energies and fluids flow freely through the liver or whether it is dense and more solid that it ought to be. If I detect the latter in a client, even if they are not noticing liver problems, I allow my energetic hands to extend way beyond my physical ones and sink deeply into the organ and listen to its messages, the reason behind its density. I may also ask the client a simple, open question about how they deal with anger. Once an energetic and/or physical, emotional, mental, or verbal connection has been made, the client's awareness and intention automatically move in the direction of exploring the issue of anger. Once we've reached that point, healing can begin.

Joanna disclosed that she had been sexually assaulted at 14 years old. The traumatic experience had been unexpressed and suppressed for decades. For decades it had been lying dormant. Not a word had been spoken about the event. Not a word had come up from the depths of her traumatized sexual organs for her throat and mouth to help her release. Her internalized, inaccessible anger was apparent during our first session. Suddenly, the emotional dam burst during the second session and her vocal cords were liberated. Yelling and sobbing and crying and shouting and raging for about quarter of an hour released the energetic block.

Josh's anger had turned inwards. What she revealed about her childhood indicated situations where rage seemed utterly justified but suppression had been the easiest way out in order to, in the short term, keep the peace. During some of our sessions, emotional outburst followed emotional outburst. Rage, grief, and anger burst out after decades of emotional imprisonment, and her cancerous liver reduced in size, visibly and palpably.

In Naomi's case, pain and rage towards her parents over events that had been forced upon her years earlier had not been uttered but stored instead, and that anger had turned inwards and festered. She came across as headstrong during our first treatment, and her emotions were locked away. At a later stage of our work together she managed to let go of the anger that had been stored for years, and once Naomi allowed herself to fully lose control, her body was forced to totally surrender to the erupting waves of emotions, yelling, shaking, and banging her fists on the treatment table.

In these examples, clients talked about fear, grief, and sadness, but anger was barely ever mentioned directly. The verbal and emotional avoidance of bottled-up anger was obvious, and the healing work we did together was instrumental in unlocking what had been suppressed. Basically, energies flow with more strength and purpose throughout a client's physical and energetic body than in normal life. In healing terminologies we call it "raising the vibration". Sometimes, I push the energy by increasing the force through my hands when I sense that the client is ready for the emotional dam to burst.

If a client is not yet prepared, or professional trust between the client and me has yet to be established, and emotions erupt in an unfamiliar way, the client may feel threatened, exposed, or humiliated. When that's the case, it takes more time and effort to build rapport with the client, who already lies supine on a treatment couch in a position of surrender and trust with a certain amount of vulnerability.

Pauline provides us with a prime example of the gradual unfolding of this process of a building of trust prior to the safe eruption of suppressed anger. During our first session, emotions came close to the surface but remained as yet unexpressed. Instead, her entire body trembled uncontrollably. Unconsciously, she was clearly longing to drop the facade of decades and for all that had been denied a voice in her life to pour out. The voice took over the next day when we met, when she pounded her fists on the couch and yelled repeatedly, "How dare they! How dare they! How dare they!" After the outburst, so much stored pain and rage had been released that her entire pelvic area was aglow, including her ovaries. She looked at least 15 years younger when she left.

After spells of intense cathartic release through shouting, coughing, spitting, crying, and trembling, Pauline was able to feel her pelvis tingling with energy, an excellent sign. Healing can only occur when energy is able to flow freely through the affected area, allowing the diseased body part to cleanse itself from energetic blockages, cancerous cells, and other sources of toxicity and be revitalized.

In my introduction to Pauline's story, I express caution regarding a client's experience and expression of anger. I'd like to reiterate it, due to a certain element of fear surrounding the free expression of this emotional charge. Based upon the fear, people are hesitant in becoming angry or only allow themselves to express a "civilized" version, whilst holding back and retaining the full force. When that's the case, the person in question may feel some sense of freedom but will never experience the full-blown liberation and full healing potential of the release of anger.

It is vital to provide an environment where the client feels contained, protected, allowed, and respected so that they can go berserk, yell and make noise, flail or punch their arms and hands, and kick or stamp their feet. They need to be convinced that no damage can be done. Precisely for that reason I work at home only, using an ancient treatment table, well padded and fabricated from solid iron, and for that reason also I've had quadruple double glazing installed in my treatment room.

If and when it feels appropriate, I inform the client that these precautions have been put in place so they can express themselves freely; however, I make sure not to put pressure on the person to "perform" or give them the sense that

I expect them to erupt somehow. Still, when I inform the client of the safety network surrounding them, it does give them permission to not hold back.

When it comes to the release of anger as opposed to other suppressed emotions, I make sure to give compliments and praise after an outburst, because it can be a scary experience at first and because anger is often judged harshly in society, hence its suppression.

What I recommend if you feel that you wish to embark on a journey of healing and you feel that the expression of anger or rage may be part of it is to be sure to find a professional who feels confident in and has experience of working with this primal force. Ask them directly about this, and if the answer doesn't satisfy you, try to find a different therapist. Do not be afraid of offending a healer, therapist, or medical professional. Instead, become acquainted with standing in your power, acting and speaking and asking from your inner source of power.

If you do not feel safely held whilst your rage erupts, your already fragile sense of trust may be scarred even further, and you may withdraw deeper into your shell of self-protection and think twice about continuing the healing journey, let alone deepening it. In therapeutic terminology, this is known as "rewounding". Remember, you're in charge of your session to a large extent. You do not come for treatments to please or serve the professional; you buy their time to serve you on your healing journey.

31

Power versus Disempowerment

The word "power" is often frowned upon and generally associated with "power over". Although this can be the case, as we see in some of the client stories, clear or clean power does not imply that the powerful person in question shows an attitude of having power over somebody else for their own gain or self-worth.

When the person in question does display power-seeking behaviour at the expense of somebody else, the person in question suffers. Such suffering can be a form of subtle emotional and/or mental conditioning, gradually resulting in patterns of obedience, compliance, and reduced self-esteem. Such suffering can equally be the result of a direct act of overpowering, such as a physical attack or a sexual assault.

Naomi was worried about her mother, and it was obvious that the mother/daughter role had been reversed. The immense pain and rage she felt towards her parents had not been uttered, but had been stored in her body instead. Gradually we ventured into the trauma locked energetically in her fourth (heart) chakra. The grief over her parents' divorce that was stored there was released initially, but the reversed role with her mother was disempowering the young woman and the growing impact of her mother on her stayed lodged in her body. Disempowerment issues are stored in the chakra associated with power, the second (pubic/sacral) chakra, whilst internalized anger and rage are locked in the liver, the third (solar plexus) chakra. Naomi fit the picture perfectly. Cancer was diagnosed in all of her reproductive organs as well as her liver.

Joanna had been sexually assaulted. As a result, her right side was severely blocked, where the body had stored the trauma by not permitting a word to be expressed from her traumatized sexual organs through her throat and mouth in order to instigate trauma release. In order to start the process of release, I started to dislodge the relational cord from her second (pubic/sacral) chakra, still linked to the perpetrator, and suddenly, the emotional dam burst.

Naturally, it had been a female organ on the right side of her body that initially demanded attention: the cyst in her right breast—the breast is very much an all-female organ, and the right side is where people store issues with the significant males in their lives (see Chapter 7). This woman had been abused by a male in her most feminine essence. In Joanna's case, her trauma related directly to the perpetrator of her abuse, who had disempowered her so severely and had created an energetic cord between both his and Joanna's second chakras.

Removal of the relational cord from the second chakra became her turning point. As soon as two people have sexual intercourse (by mutual agreement or not), a relational cord is created between the second chakras of both people involved. When, as in my client's case, the cord is formed as a result of abuse, the pain, shame, rage, and humiliation are rarely fully dealt with as long as the cord remains in place. Memories and their impact can spook the abused in mind and body, often preventing liberated sexuality later in life. The second chakra is associated with power, as noted before, so a long-lasting feeling of being disempowered and victimized can result.

To the casual observer, Joanna seemed to have overcome such negativity through positivity and drive; however, she was still in turmoil and had frequent nightmares, a clear sign of a troubled inner world. It was exactly this aspect that required attention.

I urge people to pay attention to exactly these kinds of signals to prevent further, more long-lasting disruptions to inner and outer equilibrium.

32

Lack of Self-Worth

When lack of self-worth plays a role in our life, questions arise in our mind. *Do I deserve to receive attention or somebody else's time and effort? Is it worth wasting other people's time by telling my story or asking a question? Who do I think I am to think that my drawing, my painting, my poetry, my composition deserves praise or compliments?*

A self-questioning and self-criticizing pattern like this is typically the result of having been overly or harshly criticized, humiliated, or ridiculed during childhood, usually by one or both parents or siblings. The rivalry between siblings may have played a role, or the parents may have favoured a brother or sister, conveying the message that somebody else's efforts are worthwhile whereas our own are futile.

When a pattern like this is prevalent in our life, our sense of self in society is affected and our mind is often filled with comparisons in which the self is judged less successful, less competent, less gifted than everybody else. The healthy or unhealthy dynamics of the individual within society are reflected in the functioning or malfunctioning of the third (solar plexus) chakra.

During our first session, Archie became alarmed by the intensity of my breath and movements at times. I had told him ahead of time not to pay attention when high healing frequencies pass through my body. Still, out of concern for me he had placed a hand on my shoulder. This indicated to me that he lived a pattern of putting other people's well-being ahead of his own.

By acting thus, Archie portrayed a social trap many of us fall into: serving others instead of serving our own best interests. Serving the self is very often judged to be selfish. Phrases pop into our mind:

> *Others need care/love/attention/looking after more than I do. Putting myself before others is a selfish thing to do. What will he/she think if I please myself and let him/her down? He/she has got it much worse than me, so of course I must help out.*

As a result, our own needs and desires are ignored in order to do what society considers the "right" thing.

Even with Archie's precarious medical state, he still tried to look after me despite the fact that there is a clear agreement between myself as healer and Archie as client—the agreement being that he is on the receiving end of a healing session and I, in my role as healer, am responsible for my own well-being.

In Patricia's case, her efforts at friendship had been met by ingratitude on the part of those she was trying to get to know, and this had undermined her sense of self-worth. However, it hadn't stopped her from trying over and again to seek their friendship. The tendency of trying over and over again is very telling. How much effort and energy was Patricia expending in her ongoing attempts to fish for friendship? How annoyed, disappointed, even angry (albeit unexpressed, obviously) had she been when once again her overtures for friendship were ignored?

Psychosomatic diseases occur precisely due to such a sequence of events; namely, when unpleasant emotions remain unexpressed over long periods of time, it creates ongoing festering and corroding deep inside the body that leads to disease.

33

The Individual in Society

I published my first book some 30 years ago, a novel; in other words, fiction. I can guarantee that the material in this book is not fiction, and the 13 client stories and two accompanying tales you have read in Part II come straight from real life.

The links between individual clients and their physical, emotional, mental, and spiritual roller coaster rides of "normal" life on the one hand and where, how, and when cancer manifested itself on the other, are my own. You might call that part fiction. Fair enough to a certain extent, but fiction not born out of fantasy but distilled from close observation of spoken words, body language, energetic language, and physical manifestation of a psychosomatic disease.

These close observations are not written with the intention of attracting accolades and disturbing the bedrock of widely accepted scientific theories and conclusions published in medical journals. That is not my aim. Instead, I hope to raise awareness of how our lifestyle is paramount in causing most diseases. It is only from a background of conscious awareness that the average person is capable of making choices and taking steps to reduce the risk of attracting cancer.

Awareness is key, but not awareness alone. Awareness needs to go hand in hand with actions based upon that same awareness.

The examples of Libby and Evelyn I referred to in Chapter 2 illustrate how the causes of seemingly insignificant physical symptoms (grinding teeth and skin problems) need to be taken seriously and their root cause needs to be analyzed and remedied. If ignored or suppressed with medication, these underlying issues immediately affect the energetic body—the aura and chakras—and the role they play in supporting our life force.

An unbalanced life creates stagnations in the aura and chakras, which may lead to psychosomatic symptoms in the long run.

Energetically, this depletion gradually undermines the overall immune system. A body with a malfunctioning immune system creates the perfect feeding ground for illnesses of any kind, from a common cold to a full-blown cancer diagnosis.

To explore where an unbalanced life can lead, I will take several examples from the perspective of an individual and unravel their effect on the human energy field. Some elements have already been introduced in previous chapters, but a more detailed description of cause-and-effect with regard to the development of cancer may be useful. The energetic body and the significance to health of its fluctuation are largely unknown. Let's try and demystify some of its secrets.

There are as many reasons why people live unbalanced lives as there are people on the planet—at the present time, about 7 billion incarnated souls. A combination of factors will play a role for most individuals, and a multitude of overlaps may show themselves in different ways, but all are woven around a single root cause. The origin of life's imbalances literally amounts to billions of aspects of how a person is living his average daily life not according to his inner calling.

34

Compromising One's Essence

Beautiful words, you might say, but what does "compromising one's essence" entail? Our essence is intricately linked with our heart's longing, which flows, in turn, out of our life's purpose for this incarnation—yet another sentence that may make you, the reader, raise an eyebrow.

Essentially, based upon experiences in previous lifetimes, a soul is given a certain task prior to incarnation. To serve this task, the perfect set of circumstances is sought for the soul to be born into. When the perfect situation is found, conception takes place between the perfect male and the perfect female, the individual's father-and mother-to-be.

Perfection does not mean easiest option, however! It is a misconception that we knowingly choose our parents, siblings, and family. Our higher self does that in the knowledge that challenges will manifest and can be overcome by the individual. To overcome such challenges, deeply embedded in our seat of the soul, physically located between heart and throat, lies our heart's longing. What we long for most in life helps us to survive hindrances and barricades. In the process of conquering those hindrances and barricades, we gain experiences and wisdom and can grow into a state of acceptance of all that was, is, and will be, radiating inner peace, inwardly as well as outwardly.

The exhortation to "follow your heart" stems from this. Almost on a weekly basis clients or students ask: "How do I know the longing of my heart? How do I follow it? How do I know whether a decision serves my heart?" The answer: listen. This is the subject of one of the next chapters, when I will expand on the art of listening.

Let's look at a few examples of somebody compromising their essence.

The ethic of having a job, earning a living and providing for wife, husband, and children is one reason why they easily make compromises, as in Julia's case. She had applied for a job at the local educational council and would most likely be appointed. She'd felt pressurized in applying, and part of her resented her fate, having to sacrifice a huge chunk of her precious time dedicated to her healing journey.

The expectation of supporting an ill or overly burdened mother and take on the running of the household to a certain extent, including caring for younger siblings, can be another reason behind compromising. This was the case with Naomi. The young woman cared for her mother, even when she herself got ill. It was obvious that the mother/daughter role had been reversed. The role reversal added yet another dose of suppressed emotions to the already immense pain and rage she felt towards her parents when they separated. All of this lay stored in her body, internalized and unexpressed.

An apt example was when her parents had engaged in a serious argument about financial arrangements and Naomi's liver had responded instantly with the onset of renewed cancerous activity. Also, when Naomi moved overseas with her mother and aunt after our joint healing work, she had a soul-crushingly horrific time and been unable to follow through on the promises she had made in my presence to show herself self-love. Throughout the entire period we worked together, her main issue was her mother. Even on her deathbed, Naomi reminded everyone to look after her mother. She remained incapable of reversing roles and allowing herself to be the daughter of her mother.

Patricia never complained when growing up. She agreed with virtually everything, cared for her younger sister, and did chores without being asked.

Another issue during childhood is having to live up to parents' expectations during the school years in order to secure a place at a prestigious university, get a good job, and start a well-paid career with all the trimmings. However well meant by parents, these types of demands more or less force a person into an attitude of self-sacrifice or they may ever so kindly be manipulated into that role.

Self-sacrifice is nothing more than sacrificing our essence, our heart's longing, our life purpose, for the sake of . . . For the sake of what, exactly? For the sake of too many facets to mention here, but I think you get the gist. Inwardly, the person knows they are compromising, sometimes consciously, but is choosing to or being forced to grin and bear it. Sometimes, it's an unconscious urge, an unspecified rumbling of discontent, often without being able to precisely put one's finger on its cause.

A wide range of psychosomatic symptoms can be the result of compromising one's own essence:

- **Grinding teeth.** Leading to tension in the jaw, gums, and neck (possibly causing headaches and migraines). Chewing food, a first step in the digestion process, can be hindered due to corrosion of teeth.

- **Digestive problems.** Partly as a result of teeth grinding, digestive problems can follow, starting with something as simple as overly frequent hiccups, acidic reflux, indigestion, and constipation, and turning into stomach ulcers or other more serious ailments, including cancer.

Ronald, for example, struggled with difficult-to-digest emotional baggage, exacerbated by his self-imposed, guilt-laden attitude to life, and a scan showed a thickening of the stomach lining and an affected duodenum.

The various emotional issues stored in the body often lead to an ever-so-gradual restriction in breathing, which again can lead to digestive issues. First and foremost, a constricted breath can obviously lead to a gradual reduction in elasticity of lung tissues, because the organ no longer expands to its full capacity. Breath brings energy. Restricted lung capacity limits the flow of both oxygen and energy. Its limitation weakens the organ's immune system, making lungs more sensitive to maladies like the common cold, bronchitis, infections, and cancer.

Digestive problems can also arise from restricted breathing. We humans spend a large part of our daily lives in a state of tension and fear, and we hardly notice our shallow breathing and restriction of air flow. Moving through life with a stifled breath has become the norm. Breath fills, expands and empties, contracts both lungs. Each time the lungs fill and expand, the diaphragm is pushed downward. Each time the lungs empty and contract, the diaphragm is pulled upward. An optimally functioning diaphragm stimulates the digestive organs directly below—the stomach, liver, kidneys, and adrenal glands. When breath and diaphragmatic flow are restricted, these organs no longer receive the necessary stimulation and digestion is compromised, which can lead to the malfunctions mentioned above.

Therefore, a gradual corroding effect on respiratory and digestive organs is to be expected when fear and tension remain in a person's physique for a prolonged period.

Remember, as soon as you make decisions and act against your heart's longing, against your own needs and desires, you betray yourself. In that light, what I often recommend to clients and students: *Try to be your own best friend. If, on top of that, you remain good friends with some other people, that's a bonus.*

35

Suppressing Emotions

The idea of suppressing emotions needs no further explanation. I have not come across anyone who does not at any given time suppress his emotions, myself included.

Gradually, more pennies dropped for Patricia in how she had been conditioned within her original family to please, to adjust and to comply to what other family members wanted or expected from their daughter or sister without taking into account who she herself really was and what she really craved for. The girl and now the adult woman had lived a more or less entirely disempowered existence without expressing any of her discomfort.

The suppression of unpleasant emotions, such as anger, greed, envy, or jealousy, is socially appreciated and valued, but more easily ignored when pleasant emotions, such as joy or happiness, are suppressed, which also wish to find an outlet.

How often do you see somebody skipping along the road or across a zebra crossing in a carefree way? It's something we might see a child do, before quickly being reined in by a responsible adult in an effort to teach the child social norms and values, in the process, stifling the child's spontaneous wish to express happiness and joy.

How often do you hear somebody singing or whistling on the street or in a shop? Rarely, is my guess. At least, I don't. The only person I hear singing or whistling in public is me at times, causing interesting looks to flow in my direction. Some people smile encouragingly, possibly recognizing inner urges of their own that they suppress. Some cast a quick glance of irritation in my direction. The vast majority, though, ignore the culprit altogether.

Singing, laughing, and dancing enhance a positive mood, liberate conditioned stuckness, stimulate energy flow, and release endorphins (happy hormones). Even faking a good mood and singing, laughing, and dancing when feeling down or depressed releases endorphins. The cells in our body remember the positive impulse and react accordingly. Laughter Yoga was created around this phenomenon.

As noted above, it is more widely accepted for unpleasant emotions to be suppressed. In general it's deemed inappropriate behaviour to burst out in anger or in tears in company or in public, leading to thoughts such as: *What will people think of me? Are my emotions justified? Am I hurting or burdening the other person or people with my outburst?*

The most common choice is to control the emotion and not run the risk of being judged by others or avoided at the next encounter and ostracized by friends and family or the workplace. So we think: *Better pull myself together. Don't be so silly. Grow up. I need to act my age for once. I need to put on a brave face. I need to swallow what is on the tip of my tongue.*

Familiar phrases? Have you heard people use them? Have you used any yourself? I bet your answer to all of these questions is a resounding yes. It isn't always appropriate behaviour to express the full load of your emotions. At the same time, who decided the inappropriateness of behaviour? To whom do or did you give away your authority?

Julia's mother had done her best to come between her and her father up to the point that when he passed away, Julia had not been allowed to attend his funeral. Sorrow and guilt were still embedded in her heart. A rich relational cord between father and daughter was evident. In our sessions, whenever she grieved for her dad and ranted about her mum, the cord became brighter and brighter, shedding the baggage of decades.

Chapter 23 relates a story about a client who scheduled an appointment with me after receiving a death sentence by her oncologist. Her aim was to try to lengthen her life and heal but when she booked sessions, her immediate worry was, "My husband will not be happy with it." I could see that, given the state of her marriage, if she followed her husband's wish, she would most definitely die within a couple of months. It was a form of conscious suicide. I wondered at the time, how many women commit suicide like this in order to please their partner, husband, children, parents, or friends; how many men, for that matter?

The phrase "I need to swallow what is on the tip of my tongue" directly references the physical aspect of our language. I invite you to check your everyday language for phrases that refer to a body part. Did you ever wonder why that specific piece of anatomy is mentioned in that specific context? Does a correlation exist? Nothing happens by accident. No word is spoken by accident. No phrase is used by accident.

Sylvia said to me, "I don't have the guts to make the drastic decision to break with my second husband" and called her situation "gut wrenching". When she was diagnosed with cancer of the rectum, her guts were playing up for real. The message her body had presented her with almost a year earlier had gone unheeded.

If an emotion is on the tip of your tongue, it means it is ready to be uttered. But since social convention may deem its expression unfitting at that particular moment under those particular circumstances in that particular company, it remains where it is—on the tip of the tongue—and travels no further.

The fact that the emotion is being suppressed can make it feel heavier and larger than it really is, and it grows out of proportion in the person's mind. *I wish I'd said it more directly. Why can't I be more assertive? If only I had been quicker off the mark. I so wanted to tell them where to go and where to stick their remark.*

That was true in Joanna's case, whose inner world revealed a far different picture from what she tried to convey to the outside world. This was symbolized by years of frequent nightmares. Decades of holding her innermost emotions back had doubtless contributed to her becoming ill. Her internalized rage was apparent during our first session. It was brewing in her pelvic area but had no outlet, no voice, and her jaw and shoulder girdle held on tightly.

What the civilized person is stuck with is the inner nagging, corroding, constant mulling things over, which creates a lingering inner tension—a tension residing in just that section of the body, or nearby. If we make a habit of not speaking our truth, the area around the tongue, the mouth, and the throat tenses up, and the aura becomes less vibrant and creates energetic blocks. As we've seen several times before, a less vibrant aura leaves the person open to the onset of illness.

Ronald was a classic example of the disease and its origins, which arose from long-term festering of emotional baggage.

As a reminder, the ailments related to suppression of emotions include: reduction of taste or smell, frequent sore throat, under- or over-functioning thyroid, grinding teeth due to a tightening jaw, and problems with the oesophagus. If initial symptoms are not dealt with by removing the root cause, more serious illnesses can slowly develop, including cancer.

36

Self-Blame and/or
Self-Chastising

What lies at the root of self-blame or self-chastising? The answer is a simple five-letter word: guilt.

By judging oneself guilty, there is a sense of deserving punishment. The foundation for this partly lies deep within the doctrine of the Christian church: sin not and you go to heaven; sin and you go to hell whilst burning in eternal fires.

Millions upon millions have been spoon-fed that powerful idea and live by the notion that a wrongdoer deserves to be chastised. What is wrong? What is right? According to whom? According to whose standards? Purely according to the holy book or the Ten Commandments? What about the holy book of the Muslim religion or the scriptures of Buddha or the various offshoots of Christianity, each preaching its own set of laws to abide by? If we dare question laws of wrong or right in a broader light, where does it leave the righteousness of sin, guilt, blame, chastising?

This is the line of questioning I take when a client feels burdened by guilt and exhibits an undeserving attitude. Such a belief covers multiple aspects of life, all of which make them feel undeserving—undeserving of taking up space, time, and attention; undeserving of experiencing joy, pleasure, relaxation; undeserving of earning a decent income; undeserving of asking for a penny more than the amount they are entitled to by law. Often it even feels on a subconscious level as if the person judges himself undeserving to breathe and consume oxygen.

Every penny, every morsel of food, every smidgen of time, space, and attention needs to be earned in their mind. Receiving simply for the sake of someone else's generosity or gratitude doesn't enter the equation. Instead, giving to others is the most normal thing in the world; to be permitted to receive in return lies beyond the realms of expectation.

For a considerable number of people, the imbalance between giving and receiving is huge. Again, a temporary imbalance is okay; a long-standing imbalance, on the other hand, leads to problems.

Although giving to others is the most normal thing in the world, ever so slowly the lack of receiving becomes an issue. At first it is unconscious, but slowly, a nagging feeling rears its head: the world is not a fair place. The person feels that they are being taken for granted (*Others always take from me*). When the nagging crawls into conscious awareness, discontent sets in. The act of giving, once the most normal gesture in the world, engenders resentment and leads to emotional distortions. And therein lies the solution: If we listen to the inner rumblings of discontent and resentment, pay attention to them, and take action, balance can be restored before psychological distortions turn into a somatic or physical disorder.

As before, the physical disorders associated with suppressing resentment or discontent and one's needs and wishes for balance, include problems in the mouth, jaw, neck, and throat area.

I saw this with Pauline, a woman with breast cancer who, following our session, gained confidence in her speech. Her posture straightened, her head and shoulders became more erect, and her eyes brightened, whereas before they'd been shrouded in dullness.

The female breast is the body part related to giving, nurturing, and nourishing. Women in a caring profession (nurse, teacher, carer) or in a caretaking role within the family, often develop breast cancer if there is imbalance arising from suppression of resentment as mentioned above. Do you know of a woman who has or has had breast cancer? If so, does her career or her caring role in the family reflect this tendency?

Josh, for example, tended to bite her lower lip constantly, indicative of a female tendency to hold in or hold back verbal expression. She had developed a pattern of obeying her husband, which he encouraged. She did this mainly to keep the peace, to appease him, and to follow social norms.

Problems along the digestive tract, from mouth to rectum, can manifest due to lack of relaxation and the sheer number of self-imposed tasks and responsibilities a person takes on. The number and heaviness and duration of these responsibilities can become all-consuming; that is, too large to handle and digest and causing indigestion and heartburn, excessive flatulence, frequent spells of diarrhoea or constipation, and stomach ulcers. Once more, when symptoms are not adequately dealt with, they can result in cancer.

In Ronald's story, you'll also find illustrations aplenty.

Others' demands, and an individual's guilt over not being able to meet these demands, directly affect the relational cords in the third (solar plexus) chakra and lead to distortions in this vital energy centre. The physical region energized by the third chakra fails to receive the necessary energetic input, impacting the digestive organs, including the liver, pancreas, gall bladder, and small and large intestines. Many an ailment linked with these organs stems from precisely this imbalance.

Young Naomi received a diagnosis of cancer of the right ovary, liver, and bowel. In her case, years of suppressed anger had turned inward and festered, and when, in between two series of treatments, her divorcing parents argued over money her liver responded immediately by indicating the onset of renewed cancerous activity.

In each case, the organ to take the brunt of the imbalance will depend on various contributing factors, including an individual's emotional distortions, all of which accumulate into actual illness. If third-chakra energy input is restricted and resentment over the imbalance of giving and receiving turns into suppressed anger, the liver becomes weaker. Why the liver? Generally this organ is associated with anger and stores emotional baggage when unexpressed.

If we experience an imbalance between giving and receiving sweetness in life (love, affection, touch), a craving for sugary foods can start in order to compensate for the lack of sweetness in life, weakening the pancreas. On a cellular level, the pancreas regulates the body's sugar levels. When emotional dynamics remain out of balance for a long time, diabetes or more serious diseases of the pancreas can set in.

Cancerous cells love sugar even more than you do. They feed on it. Sugar does for cancerous cells what compost does for plants. Indulging in an overdose of sweet treats, no matter what the reason, can kick-start cancerous growth and allow it to explode out of control.

If life keeps piling on worries and circumstances feel too much to handle, the ongoing tension and stress can become too much to digest—"too much to stomach", as the expression goes. Worry, stress, tension, and the like restrict how a person breathes. Less breath means less movement in the diaphragm and less stimulation of the organs in its vicinity, including the stomach, and less movement in the stomach can hinder digestion. A variety of psychosomatic symptoms can be the result: heartburn, indigestion, excessive wind, and ailments like ulcers or cancer as a more long-term consequence.

The lists of cause and effect for cancer and other diseases can be extended ad infinitum, with many variations on similar themes. In the next chapter, we'll explore one more aspect in a person's life.

37

Disempowerment

For many people, the word "power" is filled with negative connotations. In general, power is associated with violence, abuse, attack, lack of safety, and has a fear-inducing effect. As a consequence, the majority of people shy away from power, from feeling power, from living in and from their inner source of power, so as not to be associated with any of the negative aspects mentioned above and thus, regarded as instigator of violence, abuser, perpetrator, or attacker. According to the generally accepted meaning of power, the victim suffers physically, emotionally, mentally, and/or spiritually. The average person doesn't wish to have someone else's suffering on his conscience.

What I've described above, however, is not power. The generally accepted meaning of power is crooked and misleading and is more accurately a description of "overpowering". Overpowering displays aggression; power displays assertiveness.

The difference between aggression and assertiveness is all-encompassing in its various aspects. Aggression exhibits power, with the self in central position at the expense of another. Assertiveness exhibits power with the self in central position whilst respecting another. Road rage is aggressive, for example; holding onto your space in a traffic jam and not letting anyone else squeeze past is assertive. Using intimidating or abusive language on Facebook to get your point across is aggressive; stating your opinion on Facebook whilst allowing others to have different opinions is assertive.

Assertiveness allows you to claim your space or state your opinion, because that is what you deserve and who you are and stand for as a human being amongst the seven billion or so fellow human beings. This is a healthy way of using power, of being powerful. It invites you to stand tall and walk your life's path in an assured, erect manner, with your head held high, even when that head rises above the crowd—because this is who you are, who you deserve to be, who and what you embody.

If you sacrifice your opinion or your position for the sake of others' comfort to the detriment of your own, you deny yourself healthy power and betray yourself. This leads to several outcomes:

- **Restricted Self-Expression**. Not expressing your own opinion in order not to upset somebody physically restricts your gateway for self-expression, meaning, your vocal cords, throat, and jaw. Energetically, your fifth (throat) chakra shrinks and becomes dysfunctional. After years or decades of moving through life in this way, psychosomatic symptoms occur, such as grinding your teeth or thyroid problems. Cancer in the oral area may follow.

- **Self-Betrayal.** When you do not claim your rightful space, stand your ground, and give up your space to please others at the expense of yourself, this imprints the image on your physical and energetic bodies, that you do not belong, and not belonging affects the first (root) chakra. Such a disempowering attitude to life literally uproots an individual. The root chakra energizes your whole immune system, and it is precisely that vital aspect that is being compromised. An underfunctioning immune system leaves a person vulnerable to any kind of virus, infection, illness, or disease of a body part, as a result of a weakness that has been established due to psychological, emotional, or spiritual malfunctioning.

- **Disempowerment.** A radical and traumatic cause of disempowerment is sexual abuse. The second (pubic/sacral) chakra, located just below the navel, is specifically affected by power, or the lack of it. In Western society, power is mainly associated with two phenomena: money and sexuality. Thus, sexual abuse directly impacts the second chakra, which is responsible for energizing the reproductive organs. The inability to achieve an orgasm or erection, or premature ejaculation can be a direct result, as well as sexual frigidity. Abuser and victim have established a relational cord from both their second chakras after intercourse, which can drain energy away from the victim and have a disempowering effect for years after the experience. In such cases, I do not cleanse or repair the relational cord, nor do I cut it. Instead, I remove it entirely. Why leave the residue of abuse in a client's energetic field?

This is what happened when I worked with Joanna. I dislodged the relational cord from her second chakra, which was still linked to the perpetrator of her attack. As I did so, suddenly, the emotional dam within her burst and her vocal cords were liberated. She began yelling and sobbing and crying and shouting and raging. After about a quarter of an hour, this released the energetic block. The energetic flow was reawakened on her right side, and she felt calm and at peace.

There you have it: the negative and positive facets of power may result in either disempowerment by choice or through somebody else's action and influence health. It is your choice whether to walk your life's path in an empowered or disempowered way.

Doing the latter, you betray yourself and restrict your own life force. Why would you do such a thing? To keep the peace with certain people who you think love you? If they really love you for who you are, they love and respect your stance as well as your opinion. If they don't, or if you feel you have to earn their love and attention, they don't truly love you. If that's the case, you may be better off without them and surround yourself with "real" friends who truly appreciate and accept you.

Doing the former, you automatically make decisions aligned with what feels right for you, for your way of life, for your priorities, for your individuality. Your actions will be centred and aligned in accordance with your life purpose and, basically, you serve your own soul's journey. As a result, you step forward filled with purpose, inspiration, and dedication to achieve whatever feels right for you on your path.

If this previous paragraph sounds too esoteric or too good to be true, let me remind you, it is your duty to live your life purpose. Let me assure you that this seemingly Utopian principle lies within reach—*if* you allow yourself to be empowered, *if* you use your power for your benefit, *if* you act upon inner promptings, and quit compromising, betraying, and crucifying yourself.

Do remember, please, how much energy it takes to hold back and dam a spontaneous impulse that is welling up from your innate sense of rightful self. Such a holding back is like a sea defence against rising tides and tempestuous storms, something we Dutch know all too well with over half of my country's population living below sea level. It takes tremendous investment and effort and zaps energy. The Dutch government maintains strong sea defences purely out of necessity. Annual maintenance takes a fair share out of the national budget.

It is no different with your body and energy levels, except your defences are a choice, as has been mentioned before. That choice of restricting the natural flow zaps your daily budget of energy levels. Energy utilized for damming the flow of spontaneity can no longer be used by your body for life-enhancing actions, such as keeping nails and hair shiny and strong and maintaining skin, organs, muscles, blood vessels, the nervous system, and normal body functions.

For example, Pauline's emotions lay close to the surface but remained unexpressed during our first session. Her entire body longed for release and trembled uncontrollably when it was still denied a voice. That voice took over the following day, as she pounded her fists on the couch and yelled, releasing so much pain and rage with that outburst that her entire pelvic area was aglow, including her ovaries, and she looked 15 years younger when she left.

When you empower yourself and live within the parameters of your individual flow, your chakras are open and spinning to absorb universal energies, you absorb solidifying energy from Mother Earth through your root and spiritual energy from your crown. Energetic alignment serves to maintain a bridge between Heaven and Earth, with you as an incarnate being living your life purpose during the present incarnation.

Doesn't that sound empowering? It does to me. Does it deprive anyone else of their power or energy levels? Absolutely not. Does it inspire others to follow your example? It sure does. Will that deprive you of your friends' company? Absolutely not. On the whole, people prefer to be in the company of individuals who embody a higher frequency of energy.

Have I advocated strongly enough for you to live an empowered life? I hope so. You'll benefit directly by creating a stronger than average immune system. Your near and dear ones benefit indirectly through the energies you radiate outwardly.

PART IV

How to Heal or Prevent Illness

38

Inner Listening

How do you know that your life is out of balance? The answer is simple: listen. Listen with your ears to your use of language. Do you easily use negative words or phrases? When you do, try to trace the origin of this negative programming. Who taught you to think negatively about the world, about surrounding society, about yourself and your capabilities and chances in life? Your father, who compared your school results to his own superior ones or who wished for you to embark on the career he was unable to follow? Your mother, who refused to acknowledge that you were growing up and becoming independent? Your siblings, who responded with rivalry and jealousy? Your teacher, who ridiculed you in front of classmates by having you answer questions about your weakest subject?

The belittling and humiliation of a child can have far-reaching consequences for the adult: a wish to hide from the limelight, fear of performing and being seen by others, fear of failure and disappointing those in so-called authority, pressure to achieve and please a partner. Conditioning can reduce somebody's self-esteem and hamper promotional chances, kill the inner artist or performer, make the person withdraw from public life, or remain silent and unnoticed in the background.

Do you recognize aspects of your own behaviour? If you do, I invite you to take the time and sit or lie still and trace when you first heard debilitating critique. Who said what to you? In what context? Who else was within hearing? What was the person's facial expression or body language like? Harsh? Threatening? Humiliating?

Listening to your unfiltered, uncensored past programming requires a great deal of courage in the beginning. Illusions might shatter about your family and your happy childhood. The Bible states, "Love thy father and thy mother," and most children have been spoon-fed such doctrines and many similar ones. Their validity is often not questioned and, instead, taken as gospel truth in the most literal sense of the word. If so, truthful listening can indeed shatter illusions and upend your understanding of childhood experiences and presumed safety. Maybe there was an implied threat or manipulative tactics, or issues were brushed under the carpet.

The truth can be hugely unsettling. It may mean you need to make changes and move beyond your comfort zone. Painful and scary as that may seem, denying the truth can cause long-standing battles to rage inwardly, along with them the emotional fretting, festering, or corroding I hinted at earlier. Under these circumstances, a corrosion of the internal physical world is set in motion, resulting in psychosomatic symptoms.

During the listening process, it is essential to be ruthlessly, yet lovingly, honest with yourself. There's no point in fooling yourself and pretending life is brilliant and problem-free when your inner world tells a different story. If problems are lurking beneath the surface, your inner world will sooner or later catch up with you. Yes, you can avoid a divorce, a difficult discussion, moving house, quitting a job. *Ultimately though, you can never avoid yourself. Avoidance is no remedy.*

How to Listen

How should we listen? On the surface, this may seem like a silly question. Everybody listens. Listening is an essential aspect of communication and discussion. Television, radio, concerts, theatre, cinema, and so on force us to listen in order to make sense of what is being performed or to enjoy the entertainment. This, though, is not the kind of listening I'm referring to.

The kind of listening I'm hinting at is inner listening: paying close attention to what's going on in your field of thoughts, your physical body, your aura and chakras (if you know how to perceive those through your HSP, or High Sense Perception). When you listen to what's happening inside, you get a true picture of your physical, emotional, mental, and spiritual state, whether peacefully quiet or filled with unsettling turmoil of thoughts or sensations.

What is the best way to listen to your inner self? A large variety of approaches can be used. You can sit still and follow your thoughts, feel physical sensations, and connect with emotions, whether close to the surface or deeper. Some may call it meditation. You may call it that or simply call it sitting still and connecting. Which word or phrase you use to typify your action is unimportant. What is important is that you take action.

How long should you sit still? Try to sit as long as feels comfortable without putting pressure on yourself, although, if you become uncomfortable, I advise you to check why. It may be an avoidance tactic, in which case, try to lovingly remain sitting still and connecting with yourself. Remember, your aim is to avoid avoidance, to no longer fall victim to it. Throughout the process, remain gentle with yourself, as gentle as you would be with a butterfly.

You can use a writing technique of sitting in a quiet space with pen and paper and allow the pen to register every fleeting thought uncensored. Why censor anyway? You write for yourself, with yourself, and only you will read what you've written. Several hours or days later, read it with an open mind, and notice if you detect a recurring theme, a spiralling and repetitive pattern, or have you surprised yourself with what you've put on paper? Look out for and pay attention to this, because it is what makes the exercise useful.

You can draw or paint whatever wishes to be expressed from your inner creative well. Again, try not to censor or criticize or limit yourself in creative expression. Maybe you yourself can make sense of your end result. Maybe you need to ask an expert to help with the analysis. If so, connect with an art therapist, and book one or two sessions for support. It is often not necessary to commit to a long series of sessions—a couple of sessions, a period of creating the next batch of drawings/paintings, then another one or two appointments. That approach will not cost you the earth but will bring you closer to yourself.

You can seek the support of a counsellor or therapist. Make sure you choose a person with whom you click so that you have a comfortable working relationship. Again, there is no need to directly commit to a long series of sessions. Sometimes, a few sessions suffice to help you over a hump in life. There is nothing to stop you from returning several months or years later when the need arises.

An energetic healer can also help you listen by clearing and cleansing your energetic body and revitalizing the energy flow and perceiving the state of your aura and chakras. As we have seen in the stories from this book, this type of work offers clarifying insights into where, why, and how your energies are becoming stagnated and what actions you can take to maintain balance.

You can ask family, friends, or colleagues for feedback on how they see you. If you choose this approach, do please realize that they may not feel altogether comfortable with your request and choose not to reply truthfully. People in your inner circle often have a vested interest in staying on good terms with you and, therefore, avoid honest feedback. Honesty is ultimately what you're after, not avoidance.

Try to be as creative as you can, and explore different kinds of inner work. Enjoy becoming acquainted, even befriended, with yourself on a more intimate level than listening if you feel drawn to do so, as long as you search for truth. Enjoy the process of growing into your own best friend.

39

Go Forth and Search for Your Truth

The World Wide Web, with its search engines and social media, has made knowledge available to the masses at the touch of a fingertip. Previously, news reports, with all their truths and untruths, were in the hands of whoever owned newspapers and broadcasting stations and was able to influence or manipulate the viewer, the listener, and the reader.

Internet access reduces the power of the mainstream media and reduces the authoritarian role of governments and the medical profession. The patient can, if they choose, explore whatever else may be available besides the diagnosis and prognosis of the medical specialist and their advice about further treatments. I commend to you Ty Bollinger's documentary series *The Truth about Cancer: The Quest for the Cures Continues*, available to watch online (https://www.gaia.com/series/truth-about-cancer-quest-curescontinues).

It is beyond the scope of this book to list everything out there, together with all the pros and cons, as such a list is never complete and changes constantly. The search for a cure for cancer has been a dynamic field of exploration for decades and will remain so for the foreseeable future. In my opinion, the cure for cancer and its prevention will involve a combination of therapies that address every realm of life: physical, emotional, mental, and spiritual aspects. If these four realms of human life are in balance, the person lives, breathes, and exists on a higher frequency of energy.

This is exactly where Dr. Rife's successful scientific approach meets energetic cellular healing. Dr. Rife managed to cure 100 percent of his terminally ill cancer patients through the application of a high frequency of energies. Can the onset of cancer or other illnesses be prevented through people living in a more constant state of a high energetic frequency? I believe so. Prevention and cure can both be instigated and stimulated by applying the right dose of energy. The combination of applications and its effect on the person can be summarized in two words: *Immune System*.

We human beings, as living organisms, come into the world fully equipped for life. Apart from an imprint based upon the experiences from previous incarnations (if our soul evolves from lifetime to lifetime, which is my belief), we are born into a physical body, surrounded by and interpenetrated by a uniquely individualized aura and chakra system—in essence, a healthy start. An essential part of the healthy start is our innate capability to fight off invasive phenomena, such as viruses, bacteria, insect bites, splinters, and so on. Our immune system tries to maintain our health so that we can procreate and keep the species Homo sapiens in existence.

An "innate" capability means that this is a capability we are born with. Because we're born with our immune system (it hasn't arrived as a new toy or tool), and because it's not something physical we can see or smell or touch, as such, people generally are not aware of it and take for granted that it simply does its job and performs its tasks. The concept of "taking for granted" is in this respect a scary phenomenon. When something is being taken for granted, there's no need to feed it, maintain it, or look after it. With regard to our immune system, the tendency to not look after it is frightening.

Health Is Our Most Precious Possession

Without health, our quality of life is under threat. Without health, we're unable to adequately nurture and nourish relationships. Without health, we're unable to enjoy any of life's pleasures. Without health, worry and concern can become the norm. Without health, daily activities may need to be scheduled around appointments with doctors, consultants, clinics, and hospitals.

With health, though, it is easy to forget that our body is in flux, constantly working to keep us balanced and healthy. With health, it is easy to forget that we are our body and that this body needs our active participation in the upkeep of our immune system.

When people are asked whether they prefer to remain healthy, the reply is an unqualified yes. But when I ask clients what they do to look after their immune system, more often than not the initial response is a look of wide-eyed surprise. The links among health, unhealth, immune system, and self-responsibility are missing in most people's minds.

Your Immune System Is Your Responsibility

To what degree are we responsible for our immune system? What basic actions do we need to take? Does a half-hour walk twice daily to walk the dog suffice? Does an apple a day really keep the doctor away? Do vitamin supplements do the trick? Does the weekly fitness class keep the body in good shape? The answer is yes and no.

All of these initiatives assist the immune system and add something positive. Walking the dog and a fitness class promote physical activity, tone muscles, increase lung capacity, expand the diaphragm, and stimulate the digestive system. Vitamins in fresh fruit and vegetables or in supplements add building blocks to the physical body that are necessary for cell regeneration. Thousands of other positive activities can be added.

This brings us to one of the essences of energetic cellular healing: the regeneration and growth of healthy cells as building blocks of the physical body. To enhance healthy cell growth and the immune system, further and more varied initiatives are needed, incorporating every aspect of our being: physically, emotionally, mentally, and spiritually. In this way, our entire chakra system is stimulated and opens to receive the necessary, health-enhancing energies from our surroundings.

We've seen in the client stories in this book, and the different ways I've analyzed them, how our energy bodies form an integral ingredient of a balanced state of health. And that brings us to the second component of energetic cellular healing: the energy body and how to maintain or repair its vibrancy.

To me, the immune system and its maintenance are the most important elements of health and quality of life, and both are undermined on a daily basis. According to a 2003 report from the World Health Organization, over 75 percent of modern illnesses, including cancer, are due to lifestyle issues—how people approach their life, their body, and their well-being.

The body works 24 hours a day to rebalance and recuperate. This is what I mean by "immune system". It is a multifaceted, all-encompassing process involving all aspects of life as a human being: physical body, emotions, thought processes, and relationship to the divine.

> Our immune system is the ongoing process of inner and outer resilience, flexibility, and adjustability of our body to maintain, recuperate, and rebalance our health.

40

Physical Aspects of Our
Immune System

Let's start by exploring our physical body. In doing so, one life-enhancing necessity stands out: food. Food delivers building blocks for cells to regenerate, meaning that healthy cells replace those that die off in a continuous process of cell regeneration. Food is not just what we eat; it is also what we drink and what we breathe.

Bodies can sustain themselves for weeks without eating. We physically weaken without nutrition, but survive nonetheless. Bodies can also sustain themselves for days without drinking. We become dehydrated physically, but survive. But bodies can sustain themselves for only minutes without breathing oxygen. I frequently emphasize the importance of breath with my clients, both because it is necessary for survival and expansion, and contraction of both lungs makes the diaphragm move up and down, thereby stimulating the digestive organs directly below.

Each cell requires oxygen in order to function. Each cell needs to "inhale" its own supply of oxygen in order to burn energy and perform its functions, a highly specialized function for each individual cell. All together, billions of cells, each with their highly specialized individual function, constitute the body, its vibrancy, and the immune system.

Oxygen and light are the two main ingredients of our immune system and are, therefore, our main food.

Each cell radiates light. A diseased cell is one in which balance has been lost, the right building blocks not supplied, and which no longer radiates light. It has become darkened and lacks the capacity for optimal performance. Compare this with microbiologist Bruce Tainio's findings, where he measured the energy frequency of cells under healthy and unhealthy circumstances.

Our bodies need infusions of light, sunlight in particular. Even though light may be unavailable due to the time of year or long-standing overcast weather, it is nevertheless available to us in the form of vegetables (and fruits), which absorb and store light in their green leaves. This is why consuming quantities of greens assists in cell regeneration and maintenance of our immune system.

When cellular balance has been disturbed consumption of vast amounts of organic vegetables can help to restore balance. Obviously, eat organic vegetables. Why would you feed yourself produce sprayed with fertilizers and pesticides? How can you expect your cells to regenerate when you feed them poisoned ingredients?

Let's now try to put some order into the physical aspects of maintaining and restoring our immune system. As stated, oxygen and light are our main food. Why? Because in order to prevent cancer from entering the body or to encourage cancerous cells to leave it, it is of vital importance to oxidize, detox, and alkalize the body.

Oxidize the Body

In order for that essential building block of our body, the cell, to be able to perform its function, it needs oxygen to burn calories and produce energy. This is a normal biological process involving chemical reactions. If oxygen supplies are insufficient, cell function will deteriorate and the cell will mutate in a process similar to that of fermentation. As a result, the cell no longer has the capacity to die off and replicate, creating an increased fermentation process and decreased function, circulation, and elimination of unhealthy cell material, and thus, an area of stagnated, darkened physical matter inside the body, the ideal feeding ground for cancer cells. So a healthy supply of oxygen is essential in order to prevent cancer and try to remove cancer.

Once cancer has been diagnosed, a reverse process of oxygenation of physical tissue may allow diseased cells to revert to healthy cells. Illness may have been caused by under-oxygenation of the body; thus, healing may be triggered by temporary over-oxygenation of the body in order for balance to be restored. In several countries, clinics offer oxygen therapy, or "ozone therapy", whereby the patient's blood is filtered through an oxygenating machine in order to increase the oxygen levels in the blood.

Another method involves the intake of hydrogen peroxide, which ought to be used with the greatest care and with the correct dosage in order to prevent damage of any kind. Please make sure to ask your chemist or doctor for advice.

Less complicated than the two options mentioned above is the increase of oxygen in the body through simple exercise and increased breath. This demands a bit of self-discipline, but it can also be fun, such as putting on your favourite music and dancing, either alone or with your friends. Do make sure, though, that you exercise in an area where oxygen is in great supply. A gym with closed windows or with air conditioning is not recommended. Ideally, exercise outside, in nature, in a park, on the edge of a lake or sea, where natural oxygen is abundant.

Detox the Body

Detoxification of the body is turning from a kind of cult found in the world of alternative healthcare into a mainstream phenomenon. Few readers will be unfamiliar with the word and its meaning, but are you equally familiar with its significance regarding cancer?

The festering and corroding origin of the psychosomatic illness called cancer, as described earlier, gradually decreases the body's circulation, throughout the body or in certain body parts. As a result of decreased circulation, the body can no longer eliminate unwanted cellular material so that it can function optimally, and therefore, toxicity increases. When this happens, it can mark an onset of cancer.

Once cancer has been diagnosed and treated medically, the regular intake of medication targeting tumours or other growths of cancerous cells (chemotherapy) increases toxicity in the body. In fact, in the first episode of Ty Bollinger's documentary series "The Truth about Cancer", he states clearly that chemo is in essence mustard gas, which was used in World War 1. When cancer cells die off as a result of medication, the dead cell material still needs to be flushed out of the body.

There you have it—three sources of increased toxicity, if and when a person recovers from medical cancer treatments: the initial psychosomatic source, the medicinal source, the elimination source. Take a moment to reflect on the impact of this trio on the human body, and it should clarify why detoxification is necessary.

The first step in beginning to detox is to stop consuming toxic food and drink. Besides requiring discipline, this can also involve breaking the habits of a lifetime. If your long-term habits prior to diagnosis have contributed to attracting cancer, it is time to change these habits, including your diet.

Cut out sugar and carbohydrates, which the body turns into sugars. Why? Cancer cells feed on sugars. If you eliminate those two ingredients, you will probably also lose several kilograms as an added bonus. Choose organic to avoid the intake of poisons from fertilizers and pesticides, and eat food that is easy to digest and nutritious, partly because physical recovery demands a lot of energy. Avoid meat and dairy, as these proteins are harder to digest. Eat fresh foods, particularly greens, and try not to overcook vegetables; steam them, instead, as this retains more of their nutritional benefits.

Drink water and plenty of it, filtered or distilled. Make sure to drink at least three litres daily. Herbal teas, such as ginger, peppermint, sage, or green tea, can aid detoxification.

Although I do not have cancer, and do not intend to attract it, most days I put ginger peels in a teapot, add a washed and chopped dandelion plant (the entire plant, including leaf and root), pour boiling water over it, and drink that concoction first thing in the morning for optimal absorption of nutrition. It costs nothing—just a bit of effort and healthy daily discipline. Considered a weed by most gardeners, dandelion is a plant that contains anti-cancerous properties. Other plants in that category are noni fruit (morinda citrifolia), chaga mushroom (a type of fungus), and marijuana (cannabis).

If you intend to take these medicinal plant products in any shape or form, make sure you purchase a good product. Buy noni juice pure and not diluted by some sort of fruit juice. For many years, I sold bottles of noni and imported the product from New Zealand (www.noni.nz). Chaga can be locally sourced in the Scottish Highlands, where the tincture is produced by a friend of mine (*www.birchboy-chaga.com*) and elsewhere, including the United States.

Medicinal marijuana has been growing in popularity, partly because of its effectiveness and partly because it has been legalized in several countries for medicinal use. On the whole, Dutch products are recommended, because they have been semi-legal for many decades in The Netherlands and as a result, the quality is often governmental controlled. You can also buy Dutch seeds and grow your own plants for juicing. Make sure to abide by the laws of the country you live in (or state, if you live in the US). My partner and I spent a night in prison and went to court in Scotland because of growing our own crop.

Other methods of detoxification involve cleansing of the digestive organs, including the colon, liver, and kidneys, by discarding waste products from the body. Your organs can benefit hugely from support of the healing process, whether you choose, for example, colonic irrigation, juicing, fasting or hydro-therapy, just to mention a few options that are available to you.

A body with cancer must deal with an increase in toxins, so it's common sense to support their elimination. The responsibility of helping the cancerous body rid itself of waste products lies with the person who has cancer. That may seem like a harsh statement, but it is nevertheless true.

Don't try to embark on such a disciplined regime alone. You may be too tired, too scared, too all over the place to get an overview of what you need to do to set up a healthful cancer-supporting programme, including what to shop for, what to cook, juicing, cleansing, and so on.

Ask for support from one or several people, and make sure that these friends or family members are able and willing to support you unconditionally, no strings attached (remember the relational cords from an earlier chapter?). You deserve their care, support, and love.

Surrendering and allowing yourself to be the recipient of loving kindness can be quite a challenge initially. My advice is simple: allow, allow, allow yourself to receive. This stage and state of allowing can be a healing aspect you need to face in order to break a lifelong pattern and restore balance in life. I will return to this later.

Alkalize the Body

It has been scientifically proven that very high doses of vitamin C, an antioxidant, reduce harmful free radical molecules resulting from oxidation in the body, a natural process that can be damaging in excess. When circulating in high doses in highly oxygenated blood, vitamin C is selectively toxic to cancer cells but spares healthy cells, unlike chemotherapy, which also kills the healthy cells required for an optimally functioning immune system. This is why it is recommended that you alkalize your body by consuming a diet high in vitamin C if you are affected by cancer. By consuming a high vitamin C diet, I mean preferably fresh vegetables and greens and fruit and not the sometimes cheaper kind of supplements. Also in this respect, please, do your research and research thoroughly, because it is your own health which depends on your actions and decisions.

Years of corrosion and festering from blocked energies in the body can lead to fermentation, a process whereby healthy cells in the immune system are gradually replaced by acidity. This prevents oxygenation of the surrounding cell tissues, creating a perfect feeding ground for cancer. To restore the balance, the increased acidity in the body must be replaced by the building blocks of a healthy functioning immune system.

German doctor Max Gerson and Dutch doctor Cornelis Moerman have done experiments and published extensively on a diet high in fruits and vegetables and its effect on healing cancer in their patients. Their recommendations can easily be traced on the internet.

Dr. Moerman recommended a diet that includes eight essential substances, namely vitamins A, B, C and E, iodine, sulphur, iron and citric acid, to which he added vitamin D and selenium at a later stage. The change in dietary habits was a main ingredient of Moerman's methodology. In typical Dutch fashion, he emphasized how economically affordable this approach was, especially in comparison to the medical and pharmaceutical world.

Dr. Gerson's recommendation can be summarized as follows: a strict organic, vegetarian diet of fruits and vegetables high in potassium and sodium; vitamin and mineral supplements; coffee or castor oil enemas.

Do you notice how strongly the theories around cancer and its possible cures from both medical doctors are overlapping?

So yes, diet is important. Many people hate the word and its associations and in the past may have tried dieting for weight loss and failed. Try to put previous failures out of your mind, because the reason for following a restricted diet this time is very different: your health. As with exercise, make it fun, make it varied, and add ingredients that tickle your taste buds.

If you like to eat curries and hate the idea of not being able to go out for an Indian meal, why not add turmeric, cardamom, cloves, ginger, garlic, and other Ayurvedic ingredients to your recipes (and juices, if you include juicing in your routine). The ancient Indian Ayurvedic tradition promotes an overall rebalancing of body, mind, and soul, of which food is a vital aspect. Again, the internet can give you all the information you require.

So yes, diet is important. Once you find your own way of both tickling your taste buds and improving your diet, try to bring variation into your disciplined regime. Dieting does involve discipline, but too strict a regime often awakens the rebel inside people (*I'm dying for a glass of wine. I could kill for a piece of chocolate. I could murder an ice cream*). Once your inner rebel whispers these phrases in your ear, don't die, kill, or murder, but by all means every now and then allow your inner rebel its pleasure.

Savouring one glass of organic red wine of a good quality on a rare occasion can be less harmful than a gnawing, dissatisfied rebel. You can find sugar- and dairy-free chocolate and ice cream.

If you're a chocoholic, I suggest 100 percent dark chocolate. According to British chocolatier Montezuma's website (www.montezumas.co.uk), 100 percent dark chocolate contains antioxidants aplenty: 100 grams contains 13,000 ORAC units, whereas blueberries (a fruit with a high concentration of antioxidants) contain 2,400 units. aIn the United States, German-owned gourmet grocer Trader Joe's sells 100 percent dark chocolate bars made by Montezuma in its stores at very reasonable prices. I guarantee that your rebel only needs a small amount of this pure and intense chocolate to satisfy its needs.

These are only a few suggestions with regard to food. Books have been written and published about the subject, and I recommend you consult those. Often they include other useful tips, websites, or a link where you can ask questions.

Stark Warning: Rest

One final physical aspect of healing that I would like to discuss is rest. Everything you've read so far is based upon my experiences with clients, what I've read, heard, watched, and studied, because I have not had cancer, don't have it now, and aim never to attract it. It doesn't mean that my body has always been fit.

A big lesson regarding the topic of rest happened for me in December 2018 at the end of a 50-kilometre cycling trip. My bicycle chain broke, I crashed, hit the road, and was hospitalized with concussion and several superficial wounds and broken ribs. That mishap had a massive effect on me, and my body cried out for rest and sleep during the three months that followed.

First, there was the jolt of fear that coursed through my body at the moment of the crash, which my body had to digest and replace with the reassurance that I had returned to safety. Second, there was the extra energy it took for my body and mind to function again, albeit to a more limited extent for a while. Third, there was the process of recuperation, during which my body needed a vast amount of extra energy to support healing. How did I know that my body required more energy than usual? As a twelve-months-a-year river swimmer I rarely feel the cold, and when I do, it's only when I'm tired. During the first fortnight after my crash I slept in a heated bedroom (unheard of), wrapped in layers of clothing (equally unheard of). My body told me what it needed, and I didn't ignore its messages, but listened and acted upon what I was being told.

True, this was not cancer. Still, the physical and psychological processes a client's body and mind go through are similar. Detecting a lump and possibly then receiving a cancer diagnosis is a shocking, life-threatening experience—this uses up far more energy than people realize. There is inner and outer turmoil following a diagnosis, but the person is still expected to function as normal, whereas body and mind actually need time and space to digest the news, potential impacts on daily life, and possible solutions. The social pressure to override this need and keep functioning as usual takes up far more energy than you might expect.

Any treatments, be they medical or complementary, require energy to integrate and shift life patterns and habits in order to be effective. Again, this process is more energy-consuming than acknowledged.

The entire process of recovery after treatment for cancer takes far more time and energy than anticipated. Patience is essential, but the patient may well experience the opposite: impatience. Impatience can easily lead to somebody forcing themself to be more active than body and mind can handle. Patterns that may have contributed to the development of cancer need to be broken and changed in order to heal the root cause of the illness.

How much time should you set aside for recovery? That's like asking, how long is a piece of string? Only you know. Your body will tell you when it feels tired and wants you to respect its needs and lie down on the sofa for a nap or go to bed for the rest of the day. Please, please, dear people, learn to listen to your body and obey its commands.

Why such a stark warning?

I've witnessed the same phenomenon hundreds of times: a client goes through a debilitating illness and recovery process, during which tiredness and temporary disabilities rule daily life. They experience a gradual return of strength, stamina, and physical capacities, feel relieved, and wish to celebrate their return to health, including now taking part in activities they have always enjoyed but have had to give up, such as long walks, bike rides, and social visits. The celebration may also include daily household tasks that were once routine for them but during treatment have had be performed by friends or family members, such as cooking, cleaning, and shopping.

This can quickly turn into an urge to once again prove useful, independent, and normal. The keyword here is "prove". When the person in recovery aims to prove something, it can so easily lead to overdoing it, moving beyond what the body is capable of and feels comfortable with at that particular stage of improvement. The body still desperately needs all of its energy to heal and cannot afford to spend energy elsewhere. So however tempting those activities might be, however much you've missed them, however much you've hated the inactivity forced upon you, try to resist the temptation to push yourself beyond your limits.

Build up stamina slowly. At the same time, celebrate every achievement, even the smallest ones (especially the smallest ones). Maybe keep a diary of every little daily breakthrough, reread it often, notice the progress, and take great pleasure in every tiny widening of your world. As I stated earlier, exercise and the increased intake of oxygen can help to prevent or eradicate cancer, as cancer cells do not like oxygen. Am I contradicting what I said in the last paragraphs by saying that? No. Moderate rest and exercise are essential, but pay gentle and constant attention to how your body responds and adjust accordingly.

CHAKRA EXERCISES

A few elements of self-care apply to all seven chakras, with a few subtle adjustments for each one. Any yoga teacher will be able to teach you specific *asanas*, or postures, that benefit the seven different major chakras. The same counts for the colour of each chakra. If you feel or know or have been advised that a particular chakra needs extra attention, aim to bring that particular colour into your daily life more consciously.

CHAKRA 1 – Root – Red

Energetically, a stronger physical body simultaneously strengthens the first (physical) level of the human aura and the first (physical, or root) chakra, which governs the overall immune system. Also, the relational cord to the earth is situated in the very centre of the root chakra, the incarnational cord. A stronger energetic connection to the earth, the physical realm, the incarnational purpose, can be a key element in survival during serious illness.

Do you wish to take charge of energizing your first chakra and your immune system? Great, you can. There are quite a few methods available, and I'm sure you will find one to suit your individual needs.

If you follow (or if you have followed) a specific yoga practice, ask your yoga teacher for one or more postures to enhance your root chakra.

If martial arts are part of your life, tai chi may suit you better and be of benefit in working with the *hara*, which combines effortless intention and grounding. I recommend reading the book *Hara: The Vital Centre of Man* by Karlfried Graf von Dürckheim to find out more about working with this part of the body.

If working with colour is easy for you, use red. Each chakra has a certain frequency connected with a certain colour, and the one for the first chakra is red. Add more red garments to your wardrobe, visualize yourself surrounded by red, and with your intention, breathe in red. If you feel artistically inclined, or always had a (secret) wish to express yourself creatively, then begin to paint, draw, or write in red.

Eat red food, specifically root vegetables like beetroot, and eat, chew, swallow, and digest in gratitude for the nourishment the earth provides for you, whilst sensing yourself merging with the abundant earth energies on your plate and in your mouth.

If visual perception works well for you, you can visualize the red root chakra rotating, spinning in a clockwise direction. By clockwise, I mean like the hands of a clock when looking at a person's body from the outside.

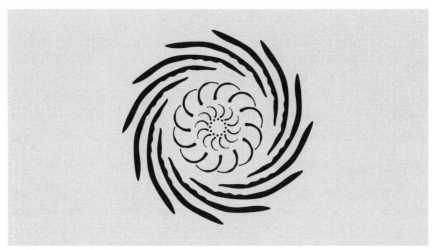

Healthy rotation of a chakra

Maybe, if living circumstances allow, begin to grow your own crops. You do not really need a garden, because you can cultivate an abundance of crops on your balcony in pots and planters. Once you become active in this fashion, an unexpected sense of purpose, vision, and creativity may begin to emerge.

People with a life-threatening illness often develop a weakening first chakra and incarnational cord. When I mentioned the healing technique of "chakra restructuring" in chapter 8, it is especially the first (root) chakra, which I restructure far more often than any of the other six, because it energizes the overall immune system. That's why I also put a far stronger emphasis on root chakra exercises than on exercises related to the other six chakras.

CHAKRA 2 – Pubic/Sacral – Orange

The second (pubic/sacral) chakra is related to power, which in Western society is related to sexuality and money. Power, empowerment, and warriorship are interrelated states of being.

In order to stimulate the sacral energy cortex, I recommend you stand like a warrior, immoveable, empowered, rooted, wide-legged, and breathe, breathe, breathe deeply and quickly. Imagine, feel, and visualize powerful orange breath entering your lungs, feeding every blood cell, and orange circulating through every artery, vein, and capillary throughout your body. Do this as long as you like, allowing it to bring you pleasure and joy.

A word of caution: make sure you remain strongly grounded throughout, and at the beginning, perform this exercise for short periods only. Your physical body needs to get used to such a strong charge of energetic power.

CHAKRA 3 – Solar Plexus – Yellow

When exercising the third (solar plexus) chakra, I recommend remaining grounded in your first chakra whilst maintaining the second chakra power stance. Chakra 3 relates to your position in society and your social surroundings. The issues stored here are guilt and shame, and the mental concepts, images, and belief systems related to these negative mindsets.

For healing to take place, negativity needs to be replaced by positivity. When you struggle with patterns of failure in your thoughts and life, of not succeeding and not being good enough, try to stand in the earlier unmoveable stance of empowerment and recite the following positive phrases, or affirmations: *I no longer need to fail. Failure is a pattern of the past. Now I can achieve whatever I wish from a solid place of power.* Feel free to use whichever phrases apply to your present situation and challenges.

In the meantime, again breathe deeply, breathing into yellow this time, the colour of the third chakra.

CHAKRA 4 – Heart – Green

When doing exercises to benefit the fourth (heart) chakra, it is essential to focus on anything that enhances a feeling of loving kindness, forgiveness, compassion, or tenderness. It does not matter who or what you focus on, as long as it brings you into a non-mental state of openheartedness. You can do this standing, sitting, or lying.

I prefer standing when I teach chakra-opening exercises, because standing encourages grounding through the first chakra and the soles of the feet. Remain grounded, and breathe slowly and deeply into the colour green, taking your time to allow the colour to penetrate your entire body. If you find it beneficial, spread your arms wide to open the heart and chest area so that it can receive the quality of love unreservedly.

CHAKRA 5 – Throat – Blue

When doing exercises to benefit the fifth (throat) chakra, note that this chakra governs the intake of nutrition and breath as well as speech. Many blocks in the throat area stem from the suppression of your voice, of not speaking truthfully, possibly in order to comply, to keep the peace, or not to sound childish, ignorant, or ridiculous. Because the suppression of speech may have caused an energetic block, speaking freely can dissolve the block and remedy the possible ailment. That is why, when writing up the exercises for chakra 3, I encouraged you to speak affirmations out loud instead of silently thinking them.

Actively using and hearing your own voice can help heal someone whose voice has previously been silenced. Singing, chanting, and reciting poetry can also assist in the opening of your throat chakra. Try not to be shy, even if it means exercising your vocal cords when nobody can hear you in the beginning and getting used to the sound of your own voice.

CHAKRA 6 – Brow – Indigo

When doing exercises to benefit the sixth (brow) chakra, you connect with celestial forces or beings. Remain grounded, in order not to leave your body energetically. It may help to place one hand over your brow and one hand on the back of your head. Breathe slowly and deeply, visualizing the colour indigo entering your body in its entirety.

If you get lightheaded, either ground a bit more or give yourself a break, drink some water, or eat a snack, and try again after several minutes. Again, your energetic and visual bodies need to get used to unfamiliar energetic frequencies.

CHAKRA 7 – Crown – Golden-White

When doing exercises to benefit the seventh (crown) chakra, you will connect with spirit and spiritual sources, whatever that may mean to you. Make sure you ground slightly more purposefully with every higher chakra you aim to open, chakra 7 being the highest. In Chapter 43, I shall discuss in detail how the crown chakra of one of my students opened instantaneously when prompted by one of his classmates to connect with his spiritual mentor, Christ.

This is one way to activate the crown chakra. Another simple way is to massage the crown of the head in a clockwise direction. Whichever approach you choose, make sure to breathe in a golden-white light, bordering on the faintest hue of violet. Imagine bathing in the acceptance and light of Christ, Mary, Buddha, or any spiritual force you feel connected with. Or imagine sitting in your favourite church or sanctuary, and allow yourself to merge with the sparkling, high frequency light of eternity.

The chakra exercises I have described can help you enhance and strengthen your energy bodies and revitalize your physical body. As noted, every chakra vibrates on a slightly different frequency, related to the different colours of the various energy vortices. Some people like to sleep under a rainbow-coloured blanket; others hang crystals in a window where the sun shines often, creating rainbows all through the room. Maybe paint a rainbow-coloured image of the chakra system, or yourself, but make sure that you use the primal colours as brightly, purely, and vibrantly as possible, because who needs dull colours?

AURA EXERCISES

Chakras are an integral aspect of our energy body. The other main aspect is the aura. These two aspects are intricately related and interwoven and influence each other instantaneously. Therefore, when you perform chakra-opening exercises, your aura benefits instantly by expanding and each of the seven specific levels strengthens as soon as you open the related chakra. Chakra 1 directly affects auric level 1, chakra 2 directly affects auric level 2, and so on. This is one very effective way of charging the entire aura, or HEF (Human Energy Field).

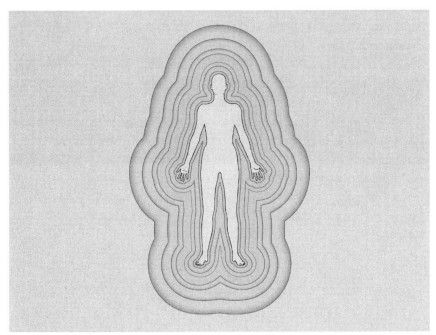

The Human Energy Field

As with the seven chakras, there are various ways to cleanse the aura. Again, it's for you to find out which approaches are easiest and most beneficial to you.

If you have a physically orientated personality, jogging, cycling, dancing, or any other form of exercise may be your preference.

If you're familiar with breathwork, position yourself so that your entire body can breathe freely, without restriction. It may be during the aforementioned chakra exercises, or you may prefer to set aside a different routine dedicated to breathing. Whatever you choose, breathe deeply into your lungs, expanding and emptying them completely, to increase the elasticity of the lung tissue.

Make sure that breathwork is a full-bodied experience. By that I mean, breathe deeply into your lower body, into your pelvis. Your lungs do not extend that far down, but if you use your positive intention, your breath will sink and sink and sink deeper and deeper and deeper.

Such a deep breath has at least two added benefits. First, the diaphragm moves up and down to full capacity and stimulates the digestive organs located directly below, namely the kidneys, liver, and stomach, and decrease emotionally stored tension in the area. Second, by breathing intentionally deep into your pelvis, you improve circulation to the reproductive organs, and again, decrease emotionally stored tension in that area.

As we've seen in the client stories and subsequent chapters, people tend to store emotional issues in the digestive and reproductive organs. The more life force, or energetic flow and freedom, you are able to transport into your abdominal and pelvic areas, the more you help shift the long-term festering and corroding effects of emotional blockages.

Other ways to look after your aura include spending *less* time on your mobile phone and computer and *more* time in nature, in the woods, and at the shore; allowing yourself to love and be loved and making love; embarking on activities that bring you joy or happiness and feed your sense of passion.

Your physical self-care influences your emotional state and may release some of your emotionally held blocks, sometimes without you even being aware of it.

41

Emotional Aspects of
Our Immune System

The emphasis of this book is on cancer as a psychosomatic illness. The previous chapters have delved deeply into this subject, with numerous examples of how an emotional imbalance can gradually create energetic blockages in the aura and chakras, resulting in a process of physical festering and corroding inside the human body and a feeding ground for cancer.

Is this process preventable? Not entirely. As a foetus, during birth, as a baby, toddler, child and teenager, we experience a huge variety of significant events that are not under our control. Many of these events are pleasant and positively influence the development of the human psyche; many are unpleasant and negatively impact that development. These negative impacts create a defence system to avoid re-experiencing similar events and the pain associated with it, as discussed in Chapter 5 in reference to Wilhelm Reich's theories around the character defence system.

The defence system harbours energetic blocks. We all have them, because our parents harbour their own defence systems and unresolved emotional baggage and behave, act, and raise their offspring from that perspective. This is not their fault. Generations before us often did not have the opportunity or the inclination to embark on a therapeutic journey of some kind. Life and life's priorities were different for them.

For example, my parents lived as children and young adults through the Second World War in the occupied Netherlands (my maternal grandparents even gave refuge to a Jewish family), and their emphasis after the war was on building security, in the shape of a safe income and a safe home in a safe environment. That was their priority after the war's lack of safety. I, as their child, have never experienced my parents' lack of safety and feelings of threat, so my priorities differ from theirs. That difference is okay, both from their perspective and mine.

My situation is not unique. On the whole, children grow up and live as adults using a different set of priorities from their parents. No blame therefore rests on your parents' shortcomings for causing defensive energetic issues, unless they deliberately made life unsafe for their offspring.

There we have it: nobody travels through childhood unscathed. Every individual develops a unique combination of emotional defences, or energetic blocks. How can you figure out what your blockages are and where you store them, why you've developed these particular issues, and how they affect your body?

The answer to this question is easy, albeit multilayered. The first step is to observe, with meticulous honesty and kindness to yourself, how certain patterns keep recurring in your life, in your decision-making, or in attracting painful situations or the "wrong kind of people".

Patterns of this kind are based upon erroneous belief systems and images. Such an image is the result of the dynamics a child has witnessed among their parents, siblings, extended family, friends, and teachers, and is often not a true reflection of reality. It is, however, a reflection of how the child, and later the young adult, has learned and been conditioned to see their social surroundings.

Evelyn, the client who I described arriving by taxi at the beginning of the book, developed a pattern of caring for other people from childhood on. Her emotions had been held in, suppressed, buried, and tucked away so thoroughly after decades of living this way that she had lost all contact with her feelings. How then to access these feelings? A first step can be to notice the pattern of caring. Once you notice and acknowledge that a pattern is operating, explore any actions that may result from that pattern that result in unpleasant emotions: resentment, feeling short-changed, a victim of circumstances, or anger.

People can embark on this journey of exploration by themselves. It takes a level of self-honesty, though, that few people manage by themselves. Often, it takes a close and truthful friend or professional to take somebody like Evelyn gently by the hand and point things out, explain gently, kindly and lovingly, the why, what, and how of the pattern and its long-term effect on the individual.

In Evelyn's case, the act of caring was a laudable one, as it was in Archie's case when he acted as substitute father for his younger brother. The laudable act creates a double bind: it provides the person with the status of being needed, of doing useful things for people and society as a whole, of being liked and respected for what they contribute *and* suffer as a result, but without consciously realizing the effect of that same laudable pattern on their own well-being.

Gently, somebody like Evelyn needs to learn to acknowledge that she is allowed to feel her emotions of anger, resentment, and feeling victimized, and that she has the right to express her emotions. The world will not fall apart if she does. If she takes a break from her caring role or quits altogether, the person she looked after will not suddenly die. People will not reject or abandon her if she begins to express her emotions. That last sentence is key, as therein often lies the main emotional block: the fear of rejection and abandonment.

As a girl, Evelyn was dependent on her parents' care. If her parents had withdrawn their care and abandoned their daughter, she might not have survived. For a child, the possibility of parents withdrawing can feel like a very real, life-threatening situation; therefore, in the child's mind, in Evelyn's mind, she had better behave the way she is expected and care for her younger siblings by taking on the caring role as a survival mechanism.

Does that sound overly dramatic? Possibly. Please realize, however, that this is the mindset, fear, dependency, and emotions of a child we're discussing, not the rational adult mind. That's one example of the unravelling of a pattern, the root cause of an emotional block, and plausible root cause of a psychosomatic symptom such as cancer.

A therapeutic setting can provide a safe and nonjudgemental environment for somebody like Evelyn to feel and even express these suppressed emotions for the first time in their life. Frequently, shyness needs to be overcome before inner permission is given to express emotions that were previously deemed inappropriate, scary, embarrassing, or humiliating.

The function of the healer/therapist is to create the safe environment, to gently and patiently encourage the client towards expression. One of the things I've found helpful in this respect is to encourage the client to breathe deeper to release an often-tight diaphragm, exhale through the mouth to open the channel of expression, and start to make sounds, any sounds, during the out-breath. Often I accompany the client in making sounds. It makes them feel less self-conscious and is encouraging.

At a certain point, we gradually increase the sound, and I encourage the client to speak any words or phrases to the person or people or institution that may have contributed to the suppression of emotions and for them to do so in their mother tongue, that is, in the language in which the holding back occurred. Although I'm multilingual, there's no need for me to understand their words—the client gaining freedom of expression is what counts. Besides, my role is to witness and support the shifts in language of the client's physical and energetic bodies.

Energetically, a more liberated emotional state of being cleanses and widens the second (emotional) level of the aura and strengthens and stimulates the second (pubic/sacral or emotional) chakra. This in turn stimulates the immune system, because energies flow freer and healthier and reach a higher frequency.

How can you work with your emotional blocks to create a more liberated flow? First of all, show compassion for yourself. Just like your family members, friends, colleagues, and neighbours, you have not come through childhood, adolescence, and early adulthood in an unscathed manner. You've been wounded at some stage, most likely at many stages, along the road.

As we discussed in Chapter 5, in order to avoid feeling the pain connected with your wound, you have developed a character defence structure, just like all the people around you; therefore, start with compassion for yourself. Defence and the avoidance of pain do not make you into a wrong person.

With compassion, acknowledge that you have pain stored that has not yet been digested. Because you have created a defence structure around your wound, around your pain, it may initially not be easy to detect your pain and its source, or sources. You may be scared of opening up the issues involved—how often have I heard a client say, "I am afraid that once I start crying, I'll never stop." Also, you may judge yourself for expressing your true feelings. If a person ought to "love thy father and thy mother" and comes to realize that some of their parents' actions were less than loving, then to express their consequent emotions out loud, with full force if required, takes courage. And support.

By all means seek support, especially initially. A true friend or brother or sister may be a suitable person. They need to be able to accept all of what and who you are, though, without the slightest judgement. As I stated earlier, such a person is not always easy to find.

When you do not know whom to reach out to in your social surroundings, seek professional help. As I have made clear, often there is no need to enter a long-standing professional therapeutic relationship; a few sessions can take the pressure off. By all means, ask the therapist to give you homework so that you can continue on your path in between treatments and after you finish your series of sessions.

If this feels too much of a stretch, risky, or possibly too expensive for you, I advise you to reread Chapter 38 on "Inner Listening". Time and again, irrespective of which approach you choose, keep returning to that state of compassion for yourself, and enfold yourself in your own loving heart. Maybe simply wrap your hands around your upper arms and embrace yourself whilst listening to the feelings that are coming up.

If, when you were a child, you had wished for somebody to listen to you and embrace you, that lack of nourishment, nurturing, and safety may well surface as pain. If that's the case, allow tears to flow, allow your voice to express your previous lack, either in words or moans and groans. You may wish to repeat a sentence, a word, a phrase, an affirmation, or mantra meant only for your ears. In the beginning, you may feel shy about using your voice to express self-love; if so, think it with all your heart and, when shyness recedes, whisper it. Do this until you're able to utter these words aloud, or until you can scream, yell, or howl your self-love throughout the woods, over the beach, into the storm.

Positive thoughts affect your sense of self positively. Positive speech affects your sense of self positively and to a larger degree, because not only do you vocalize your self-love, you also hear it.

When wounding occurs, love is absent. In order to heal wounding, infuse yourself with love, compassion, tenderness, and safety in total acceptance of who you truly are and who you have developed into as an adult here and now.

42

Mental Aspects of Our
Immune System

Emotional and mental aspects are often strongly related. The mental side of cancer's root cause concerns itself with the individual's images, belief systems, and thought patterns. In describing Evelyn's background in the previous chapter, we unravelled the interwovenness of emotion and mental aspects of our immune system.

Basically, mental concepts are not similar to emotions. They can, however be created by emotions, or the avoidance thereof. In this respect, let me revisit what I wrote about Evelyn.

Like all children, she depended on her parents' care, so if they had withdrawn that care and abandoned her she might not have survived. For a child, the possibility of parents withdrawing can feel like a very real, life-threatening situation, so, as a survival mechanism, the child thinks they had better do as they are told; in Evelyn's case, care for younger siblings by taking on the caring role. It is the mindset, fear, dependency, and emotions of a child, not the adult rational mind.

In other words, the emotion "fear" causes the image or belief system that "my survival depends on my obedience and on me complying with what is expected of me by those in authority". The opposite is also true. A person's mental concepts, images, belief systems, and thought patterns can lead to emotional reactions, or the suppression thereof.

Evelyn needed to learn to acknowledge that she was allowed to feel emotions of anger, resentment, and feeling victimized, and that she had the right to express her emotions. The world was not going to fall apart if she did. She will not be rejected or abandoned for expressing her emotions. In other words, Evelyn's image or belief system—that survival depended on her complying—made her fearful that if she expressed her emotions truthfully, care would be withdrawn. The image made her frightened and she obeyed, in the process suppressing her own emotions. In this way, people's emotions (or the suppression thereof) can create an unbalanced mindset or image and belief system, and in this way, an unhealthy mindset can lead to the suppression of emotions.

Energetically, as we noted earlier, a more balanced mental state of being cleanses and strengthens the third level of the aura, the mental level, and strengthens and stimulates the third (solar plexus) chakra, or mental chakra. This in turn stimulates the immune system, because energies flow freer and healthier and reach a higher frequency.

I invite you to read Archie's Story again, as well as what I wrote earlier about the experiment in the Chinese medicine-free hospital, where the third chakra and third level of the aura are strengthened by the repetition of a positive word to such an extent that a cancerous tumour fades away within three minutes. Yes, this is an extreme example. Still, extreme or not, it occurred and was filmed, and it can be repeated.

The three people standing around the patient's bed had been specifically trained to raise their energies to a healing frequency and maintain that frequency throughout the experiment. They chanted, "Already done. Already done. Already done." The trio held the intention in their love centre, in their hearts, that the patient's tumour had faded, and they confirmed that mentally by speaking and chanting in Chinese that the healing had been completed. The impact was remarkable, and healing happened rapidly.

Whilst you, the readers of this book, may not have special training, you can hold the patient, your father or mother, your brother or sister, your neighbour, friend, or colleague in your love centre, in your heart, whilst speaking aloud or chanting phrases like "Healing is possible." "All cancer can be healed." "Healing has happened." "The tumour can shrink and disappear." "Illness is no longer needed." And so on.

Allow yourself to be creative regarding the sentences you use and adjust your vocabulary to the person or people involved. If the patient has a strong affinity with nature, include the mentioning of trees, plants, flowers, birds, butterflies, or other natural beings of power and beauty. If the patient is strongly attached to a cat or dog, by all means include their names and their love, and maybe have the animal present. Pet's love is often unconditional and can only add to the overall atmosphere of healing and love.

If you wish to try this with several people around the bed of a loved one who has been diagnosed with cancer, feel free. As I see it, you cannot do any harm. Love and your loving intention can only do good. You may need to practise raising your frequency, through extra grounding and increasing the depth and speed of the breath. You may need to reach a certain level of experience in doing so effortlessly in order to be able to maintain the required energy frequencies. You may need to spend some time in joint silence or meditation when you perform a healing circle with other people. Jointly, you create a strong field of healing energy, which is far more impactful than the separate fields of healing of the different individuals.

Although I cannot see any harm in doing this type of healing experiment, try not to experiment willy-nilly with such techniques. Healing is an ancient and sacred art and needs to be performed with great respect. Perform the healing work in a place and at a time when you won't be disturbed. Make sure that all electronic equipment has been switched off in advance, because electronic radiation is a lower frequency than that of healing. Make sure, too, that both patient and participants drink plenty of water afterwards. Finally, give thanks to the unseen ones, the discarnate ones, who will doubtlessly be present in support, whether you sense them or not, whether you believe in their existence or not.

How can you improve your mental programming and reduce or remove blocks on the mental level? Again, by all means invite the guidance and support from a therapist who has been trained and who is experienced in guiding their clients through the maze of past conditioning. If you choose not to use the expertise of a professional and go it alone, try to follow your train of thoughts—thoughts about yourself, thoughts about your illness and your diagnosis once the illness has manifested in your body, thoughts about your chances of recovery and the path to recovery. To follow the twists and turns of your mind accurately, I recommend you seek time and space and quiet to enhance a sense of focus and mindfulness.

Once you enter such a space of intimacy with yourself, allow thoughts to wander and arise without judging them, without judging yourself in any way. Also on the mental level, try to come to a place of compassion for yourself. Most of your inner train of thoughts is not really who you are. Most of your inner voices and opinions have been planted in your mind by people from your past, mainly people from your childhood, such as parents, grandparents, siblings, and teachers. With the innocence of the child you accepted their opinion as gospel. That acceptance was not a mistake, but simply what was expected of you.

Whilst following your thoughts, try and trace common denominators, such as a word, a phrase, a statement, an opinion that keeps returning. A common denominator can be a powerful message that life has presented you with and that you keep repeating because the message has been repeated so frequently, or a specific life's event has had such an impact on you, you made the message into your own and keep repeating that message.

Pauline, for example, devoted herself to caring for her mother all through her slowly progressing ovarian cancer. She was heavily impacted by the experience. Gruesome images haunted her, and she began to believe that she too would face ovarian cancer, which did, indeed, come to pass a couple of decades later.

Although Pauline would have noticed her repetitive train of thoughts, she would neither have had the awareness nor the insight to change her way of thinking. In her case, if I had been her therapist at an earlier stage of her life, prior to the cancer diagnosis, I would have recommended that she try to notice if and when her thoughts went in the direction of overidentifying with her mother and her mother's path of suffering. At such a moment, I would have made her aware that her life's journey and her mother's life journey were two very different paths, with different directions, challenges, and possibilities.

Once that awareness settles in the mind, it is important that the individual changes the common denominator into a sentence with the opposite meaning: "I am not my mother. I am a person in my own right, travelling my own path. I do not have to take on or copy my mother's suffering. I have the awareness and the power not to attract cancer or any other serious illness."

Every time you contradict earlier conditioning, you chip away at the block of marble to allow the envisaged angel of healing to emerge. It takes patience, but with each chip a bit more of the angel becomes visible, a bit more of the unique personality begins to manifest. This chipping away at childhood conditioning influences the third (solar plexus) mental chakra and the third mental level of the aura positively and strengthens both elements of the person's energy body, contributing to a stronger overall immune system.

43

Spiritual Aspects of
Our Immune System

The physical, emotional, and mental aspects comprise our individual personality; however, spiritual aspects move beyond our individual self into the realms of spirit, faith, religion, universal trust, and the like. The physical, emotional, and mental aspects influence the first, second, and third chakras and the first, second, and third levels of the aura; however, spiritual aspects directly affect the seventh (crown) chakra and the seventh or outer level of the aura.

The energy frequencies of this chakra and auric level are much finer, more sensitive, and higher than the lower ones, and they react much faster to changes. To ignite healing on the spiritual level, a sense of faith needs to be restored where previously fear or anger or grief or any other energetic distortion may well have dominated.

Achieving this is a uniquely different journey for each individual, depending on their upbringing (religious or non-religious) and experiences that may have contributed to them establishing a source of faith or a lack of faith.

As we saw in an earlier chapter, when a chakra rotates clockwise, the energetic body draws in energy and life force, essential for the person's well-being. The seventh chakra, the crown, is the gateway to our spiritual connection and source of divine energy, including our sense of faith. When the crown chakra rotates clockwise, high frequencies of divine light enter our energetic and physical bodies.

How that can be achieved spiritually, let me illustrate with the following story from one of my classes.

As part of a Bodies of Light training exercise, students practise reading each other's chakra movements using a pendulum. During one of those sessions, a student registered that his classmate's crown chakra was closed (the pendulum did not move), despite a strong faith in and active connection with Christ. The student looked at me, puzzled. I responded by inviting his classmate to connect consciously with his spiritual mentor, Christ. Instantly, the pendulum went berserk, rotating clockwise in a massive circle, signifying the chakra opening and spiritual energies entering his aura and body, and the seventh (outer) level of the student's aura lit up and was strengthened. A strong and vibrant outer level functions as a kind of buffer zone, a filter to protect the lower levels of the aura and the physical body from negative, frequency-reducing input.

This is a telling example of how an active spiritual connection can promote health and well-being in the blink of an eye, namely my student's instantaneous, energetic reaction to my invitation. Just imagine what a more or less constant and consciously active connection to divinity (in whatever shape or form) does to your health.

Several times during sessions, I have witnessed the immediate effect a direct spiritual connection can have. On a few occasions a client with an active religious discipline went into prayer during sessions. Each time the result was awesome. Because they allowed themselves to pray with heart and soul, in total surrender to their connectedness and to the healing, energy flowed more unhindered than normal, chakras responded more effortlessly, and the aura cleansed and expanded more quickly. In a nutshell, the prayer and the spiritual activity enhanced the healing potential and receptivity of the client. Such tendencies are not limited to healing sessions. Every time a person allows for the embodiment of a spiritual connection to filter into and through his body in its totality, the immune system benefits.

I recommend that you create periods of silence in your daily routine. Let your loved ones know ahead of time that you do not want to be disturbed, or put a DO NOT DISTURB, PLEASE sign on the door and switch off your phone. This exercise may be done in either a comfortable seated position or lying down; make sure that you're warm and comfortable.

Picture, in your mind's eye, a person, animal, entity, or scene, someone, or something that is uplifting and inspires you. When you connect with your source of inspiration, breathe in its essence and allow it to envelope you and fill every cell of your body. For my student, this source of inspiration was Christ. For Naomi, it was St. Francis. For you, it may be Mary, Buddha, Sri Baba, your son or daughter, your grandchild, your beloved pet, a landscape with a mountain, lake, sunset, or some combination thereof. Your choice depends on your preference and nobody else's.

Breathe in the essence of the image in your mind's eye. Feel yourself being filled and enveloped by its exquisite beauty, and ever so gradually, allow its pure acceptance and light to fill you. Feel each and every cell of your being filling with light, filling with beauty, filling with spiritual essence. Take your time—I can guarantee that within several minutes you'll feel lighter, more spacious, and that any troubled thoughts will have lightened or faded altogether.

It may take a few tries to start to feel the full benefit, if you're not used to visualization; it will get easier with practice, so repeat often. Don't expect to reach an identical state of expansion every time, and try not to put pressure on yourself—most likely you've done that too often in the past. Remain gentle with yourself, as gentle as you would be with a butterfly, and enjoy your flight into freedom.

Each time you sense this lightness entering and enveloping you, it means that you have managed to expand your aura; that you have managed to open your seventh chakra, and possibly your chakra system in its entirety; that you have given your immune system a boost; and that you are feeding your body's cellular memory with positive healing vibes.

Try not to underestimate the long-term effect of the latter. When you're not well, it means that the memories stored in your cells are overwhelmed by negative baggage that has triggered illness. By placing your energetic and physical body on a higher, healing energetic frequency, you reduce the weight or intensity of negativity stored in your cells and replace negative vibes with positive ones. As we've seen in chapter 8, positive thoughts have a direct impact on the DNA, as well as on your well-being and on your health.

Yes, these shifts are subtle. Practically all vibrations in the spiritual realms are subtle. Nevertheless, they exist, and I strongly encourage you not to doubt the healing power of the subtle world of spirit. By the same token, if you feel changes in vibration as a result of doing these exercises, try not to doubt these changes. You're not making it up. Spirit and its energetic vibrations is as real as you are—as real as the chair upon which you sit, as real as the house you're living in, as real as the car you're driving. Unfortunately, in our modern-day society, we create very little space and time to feel, sense, let alone acknowledge spirituality and its wondrous magic.

When you allow yourself to dwell more consciously in silence, in wonderment, in purely natural surroundings, in places or buildings of worship, in sacred locations, in the company of people who inspire you, an entirely different world may open up to you. Initially unfamiliar, you may gradually discover a peace deep inside, an at-one-ness ignited by your perfect choice of surroundings or company or both.

44

Pioneers Are Often Ridiculed

In the 15th century, explorer Christopher Columbus stood on the shores of his native Italy and looked out to the horizon, where sea and sky meet. His keen eyes detected a tiny tip appearing on the horizon after a while, and watched as that tip gradually elongated into a ship's mast, complete with crow's nest, banner, and beneath that, sails, and then the bulk of the vessel became visible. The sequence made him question what he was seeing, so he decided to wait and see whether the phenomenon would be repeated a second time, a third time, and so forth. He sailed out to sea himself and watched as the coastline behind him faded into the distance. The last visible aspects were top floors of storehouses, treetops, the cathedral spire, and finally, more distant hilltops.

His conclusion: the earth is not flat but round.

This led Columbus to theorize whether it might be easier to reach the shores of Japan, China, and the Indies to the east via a new, westerly, and perhaps shorter trading route. He asked the authorities of his native Genoa for a ship and crew in order to mount an expedition to prove his theory, but was met with ridicule. The same thing happened when he put in a similar request at the Portuguese court. But Spain, the third country he petitioned, granted his wish, and the rest, as they say, is history.

Pioneers of all types are often met with disbelief, ridicule, harsh judgements, and lack of cooperation and support. If the establishment feels threatened by novel ideas and theories, this can have severe consequences for the pioneer and their work, leading to economic and/or political action against the pioneering initiative.

The same happens with regard to cancer and the search for solutions to the worldwide spread of the disease. New horizons are being explored continuously by many individuals, be they scientific researchers linked with universities, such as Dr. Raymond Royal Rife; medical doctors linked with hospitals, such as Dr. Ryke Geerd Hamer; or individuals who feel motivated to move beyond the familiar and acceptable, such as documentary maker Ty Bollinger in his 2018 series of documentaries *The Truth about Cancer: A Global Quest*, or practitioners like myself working with energetic cellular healing. For now, I wish to introduce a few of the aforementioned pioneers to you.

Dr. Raymond Royal Rife: A Shocking Truth

Cancer can be cured. This was proved scientifically almost a century ago.

Dr. Raymond Royal Rife, a scientific pioneer and genius, developed a unique and complex microscope almost a century ago. Using his Universal Microscope, he was able to observe the reactions of the tiniest micro-organisms (viruses, bacteria, and so on) and noticed whether they disintegrated or changed form under influence of specific circumstances. The device enabled him to record the precise energetic frequencies with which different pathogens (illness-causing infectious cells), normally traced in blood and/or tissues from many diseases, could be destroyed.

Throughout the 1930s, Dr. Rife carried out tests on animals in his specially designed laboratory that proved very successful. Encouraged by what they were seeing, the medical school of the University of Southern California in San Diego presented Dr. Rife and his team with 16 human terminal cancer patients with a variety of symptoms as a trial. The team was able to declare 14 of those 16 terminal patients clinically cured after 70 days; the remaining two patients were cured within the next 20 days after the team adjusted the energetic frequencies of the applied resonance.

The medical and pharmaceutical world concluded that Dr. Rife's method would be able to cure many illnesses without the intervention of surgery or drugs. However, because drugs and surgery generate money, careers, and profits, Dr. Rife's theories and techniques were hushed up and declared worthless. After many legal battles, documents of the USC's clinical trials vanished, equipment was confiscated, laboratories destroyed, one medical doctor may have been poisoned, another harassed until he left the job, and a third seemingly committed suicide.

Further attempts by Dr. Rife to make his work available to the general public were met with similarly destructive methods. In 1961, he fled to Mexico and died in poverty 10 years later at the age of 83. Profits were considered more valuable than the lives of people with cancer. Has anything changed for the better during the last century? Unfortunately, no.

On 10 April 2018, Goldman Sachs published an article entitled "The Genome Revolution" in its *Equity Research* magazine. The biotech research report, asks whether curing patients is a sustainable business model.

The potential to deliver "one shot cures" is one of the most attractive aspects of gene therapy, genetically-engineered cell therapy and gene editing. However, such treatments offer a very different outlook with regard to the recurring revenue versus chronic therapies. . . . Whilst this proposition carries tremendous value for patients and society, it could represent a challenge for genome medicine developers looking for sustained cash flow.

In other words, business and profit before cure; money before health.

The article does not mention cancer. Still, it is a well-known fact that the illness helps to keep a multi-billion pound/euro/dollar pharmaceutical industry afloat. When a new drug has been developed to possibly lengthen people's life if taken on a daily basis for the rest of the patient's life, who benefits? Maybe the patient benefits to some extent when side effects are not too severe. Maybe friends and family benefit to a similar extent when they don't see their friend or sibling suffer unduly due to side effects. The company producing the drug and its shareholders are certainly beneficiaries. As long as healthcare and production of medication are profit enhancing, prioritization of patients' interests cannot be expected.

Dr. Ryke Hamer

From 1963 until 1986, Dr. Ryke Geerd Hamer held a German licence to practise medicine. His motivation to explore the cause and cure of cancer was based upon his own experiences—he had himself developed testicular cancer after the sudden and violent death of his son. He sensed the two events were strongly linked and so began research.

Over the years, he was able to work with and observe thousands of patients, both on a physical and emotional level. His research showed how emotional conflict ended up manifesting as physical disease, how the whole disease process can be understood as an adaptive mechanism, and how patients can heal. His well-documented work has been a valuable contribution to modern medicine.

According to Dr. Hamer's website, German New Medicine:

> When we have a shock, a disease process can be initiated. However, when the biological shock is resolved, this activity will come to a halt. This activity will take place on the organ, and depending on the particular cellular structure that was affected, this activity can either develop into a growth (tumour) or it could begin to degenerate tissue on an organ.
>
> The location of this activity on the organ is determined by the exact nature of the conflict.

> When this conflict activity stops, the body will naturally go into
> 'healing mode'. However, this is also when approximately 60 to 70
> percent of our diseases will be diagnosed, and that includes some
> cancers. On the other hand, when a growth develops during conflict
> activity, it will stop growing and either lay dormant or degrade
> when the biological conflict is resolved.

That's quite a statement, isn't it? However, it is a fact, and traditional medicine has already observed this. They just couldn't explain it until Dr. Hamer began to look for answers. As a matter of fact, approximately 50 percent of all cancers that grow during conflict activity are already dissolved and dormant at the moment of cancer diagnosis.

This implies that the cause of cancer, as with many other illnesses, lies in events (conflict activity) that are experienced as traumatic, based upon the perception of perceived or actual danger. If such a "biological conflict" is resolved, the body enters a healing stage and health can be restored. The implications of this according to Hamer: medical intervention is often unnecessary, even for serious diseases.

I described in "Julia's Story", how cancer appeared and killed a woman in our town within a few days after she had been robbed in broad daylight on the street. Her autopsy showed an abnormally aggressive spread of cancerous cells all over her body whilst she had been perfectly healthy prior to the crime. This story illustrates painfully the correlation between experiencing trauma and the onset and spread of cancer as advocated by Dr. Hamer.

Dr. Hamer's license to practise medicine was cancelled in 1986, and his methods judged a danger to the public. The approach seemed too controversial. Too pioneering? Sailing too far beyond a safe horizon and opposing the establishment, perhaps. Universities in Germany and professional oncology organizations in Germany and Switzerland concluded that Hamer's work lacked scientific methods and his arguments did not back up his experiences or theories.He definitely is not a person without controversies.

The case of six-year-old Austrian girl Olivia Pilhar speaks volumes. The girl suffered from Wilms' tumour, and her parents brought her to Dr. Hamer out of fear of the painful conventional therapy. Dr. Hamer diagnosed no cancer, but instead several conflicts. They fled from their native Austria with their daughter to Spain to escape the Austrian government, which had removed the parents' rights and control over Olivia. After intervention from the Austrian president the family returned to Austria, where the girl received conventional treatments. In the meantime her health had deteriorated significantly, but she survived.

Also his anti-Jewish conspiracy theories are hardly salubrious. Dr. Hamer saw his method as a "Germanic" alternative to mainstream medicine, which he claimed is part of a Jewish conspiracy to murder non-Jews. As a result of these controversies over a period of a couple of decades, he was arrested and banned from practising in several European countries, and in the end, sought exile in Norway, outside EU borders.

Although these are serious black marks against a practitioner, I would plead against throwing out the baby with the bathwater. When I first encountered Dr. Hamer's observations and theories about cancer patients and their reason for attracting the condition through trauma or psychological imbalances, and a potential cure, I distinctly remember feeling that I had encountered a kindred spirit.

One controversial aspect is likely to have been Dr. Hamer's stance on conventional medical procedures like chemotherapy and radiation, which he believes do more harm than good, due to the destructive way they work: attacking and destroying healthy as well as cancerous cells.

In fact, in his series *The Truth about Cancer*, Ty Bollinger interviews quite a number of medical professionals who agree with Dr. Hamer's views on chemotherapy. To quote but a few:

DR. SUNIL PAI: "90 percent of physicians, especially in oncology, will not undergo chemotherapy for themselves or give it to their wife or child."

DR. ALEKSANDRA NIEDZWIECKI: "Chemotherapy uses the most powerful toxins known to humans. It is being given to kill cancer cells, but it also kills healthy cells and damages organs, which makes recovery from cancer almost impossible. Instead of curing cancer, we are generating new cancer."

DR. BEN JOHNSON: "It is estimated that by 2020, half of cancer cases will be medically induced by drugs or radiation. So our medical establishment itself will soon become the leading cause of cancer in the USA."

DR. BOB WRIGHT: "97 percent of people who undergo chemotherapy are dead within five years, according to the *Journal of Oncology*."

If you wish to hear more reality checks from medical professionals about what is generally being accepted as normal, albeit often harmful, practice in the medical profession, I definitely recommend Ty Bollinger's valuable contribution to the global cancer discussions.

Back to Dr. Hamer. As you can see, he most definitely is not alone in his criticism of the widely accepted medical approach towards cancer. My sense is that the pioneering aspects of this man's work may well turn into one of the cornerstones (adapted and fine-tuned, however) of the medical approach of the future.

Dr. Stanislaw Burzynski

Another revolutionary practitioner when it comes to finding a cure for cancer is the medical doctor and biochemist Stanislaw Burzynski. His video "Burzinski, the Movie: Cancer is Serious Business" is worth watching and readily available on the internet.

Of Polish descent, Dr. Burzynski moved to the United States in the 1970s and discovered a nontoxic, gene-targeted cancer medicine. It might well have changed the way cancer is treated were it not for the fact that his discovery was suppressed by the US government. Dr. Burzynski and many of his patients had to face a 14-year-long legal battle before the FDA finally approved clinical trials for his methods.

Dr. Burzynski discovered that antineoplastons, nontoxic peptides and amino acid derivatives, function as a switch to turn off cancer, suppressing genes as well as turning off oncogenes (cancer genes). Antineoplastons actively attack cancer genes and stimulate the function of molecules, which deactivates cancerous cells. His terminally ill patients outlived those other cancer patients who only received medically prescribed drugs.

Dr. Burzynski's methods had better outcomes than all other available conventional medical treatments, and this is undoubtedly why he faced strong opposition. Why suppress the truth of a cure for cancer? I suspect that the answer is the usual one: the financial profits of the pharmaceutical industry and its shareholders are more important than the health of ordinary people and their family and friends reliant on conventional medicine for a cure.

To my knowledge Dr. Burzynski is still practising and his clinic (*www.burzynskiclinic.com*) is in existence as I write.

Conclusion

My Wish for the Future

As with any other psychosomatic disorder, treatment for cancer needs to address the following elements: work on the physical body, release of suppressed emotions, a positive mindset, and a spiritual awakening. When healing only occurs physically, it's like putting a sticking plaster over an infected wound. Underneath the plaster, the wound festers and corrodes, gradually affecting a larger area of the body and turning from a mere surface wound into a poison affecting the person's insides.

Our energetic bodies respond to either a positive or a negative mindset, to either pleasant or unpleasant emotions, to either an inspiring or an uninspiring connection to the divine. And they do so in the blink of an eye. That response can lead to a change in the physical body.

Positivity, pleasure, and inspiration, as we've seen, can retain or regain health and well-being and stimulate the overall immune system. Negativity, displeasure, and lack of inspiration can undermine health and well-being, invite the onset of disease, and weaken the overall immune system. The same happens in relation to cancer.

In "Julia's Story", you read how a local woman's body became riddled with cancer instantly after having been attacked in the street. Removal of cancerous activity can occur equally quickly, although such an occurrence is exceptional. Still, such an instant healing shift lies within the realm of possibility with a hopeful and positive mindset, a focus on pleasurable emotions, the right physical conditions, a supportive social network, and an inspiring connection with the divine, which raises the individual's energy levels.

The fear-based approach to cancer favoured by the medical world, and society in general, largely shuts down the chakra system and creates density in the various auric levels. This blocks positive healing energies from entering the physical body at those important energetic points just when the body needs healing energies more than ever before.

The hope-based approach, in which a patient is empowered and supported as they explore how to proceed on their individualized healing journey, strengthens the chakra system, keeps it open, and maintains a more vibrant and clearer aura. As a result, revitalizing energies are automatically absorbed.

This support can come not only from family and friends but support groups, and especially from practitioners within their specific field of profession, be they medical or complementary.

Just a word here about professional support.

Once a client seeks professional help, whether from a medical doctor or a healer, I see it as the responsibility of professionals, whether complementary or conventional, to support the patient in unravelling the inner imbalances that created the energetic blocks in the first place and contributed to bringing on cancer. If the consulted professional is unable to provide this support, in an ideal world, the consultant is responsible for directing the patient to a colleague, or an organization where this individual support can be found; that includes if this colleague or organization is part of "the other approach" to healthcare.

In our profession as (health) consultants, we need to bear in mind that we work for the benefit of the patient, and this includes urging patients to become responsible for managing their health. If I am unable to assist clients further, for example, I refer patients to colleagues with more specialized expertise who can support patients in delving deeper into their health issues. I would hope that this would work both ways between the medical profession and the healing community. It goes without saying that there must be open lines of communication and free exchange of information among the various professionals and professional organizations and individual healers, with the aim of improving outcomes for our patients.

Together with their support system, a patient can create their own scheme of independent self-healing according to the following mindset: *I have created cancer by ignoring my true self. I can heal cancer by acknowledging my true self and making choices that truly serve me.*

A similar mindset and sense of self-responsibility holds the key towards prevention of cancer: *By acknowledging my true self and making choices accordingly, I can prevent attracting illness, including cancer.*

I invite you to feel into this concept for a few minutes. Now compare this to a concept reflected in newspaper headlines, quoted in an earlier chapter, stating: "Two-thirds of adult cancers largely due to bad luck."

I invite you to feel into the differences in these contrasting concepts for a few minutes. Do you notice how your body, your emotions, your mind, and your spiritual connection are different depending on which concept of health you focus on? Which concept creates a more positive response inside you? Which concept makes you breathe with more ease? Which concept makes you feel less restricted or more liberated? Which concept makes you feel empowered, in the driver's seat of your own life's destiny? Which concept makes you feel less like a victim of circumstances?

To me, it is simple self-explorations like these sparked by simple questions that can help you find your individual road map to health, one tailored to your needs at this particular stage of your disease or healing process.

If you feel that such an approach lies beyond your reach, maybe because you're unfamiliar with inner work or because of a recent cancer diagnosis you can't think or feel straight at present, then search for guidance and contact a therapist or counsellor. As discussed earlier, just two or three sessions can assist you along the road of self-exploration, self-discovery, and self-empowerment towards healing.

When you start down the road towards self-determination, you will be amazed at what you uncover. First, what the body has stored as traumatic experiences. Second, the number, depth, and power of suppressed emotions. Third, what the mind has stored in habitual thought patterns that have led to such alienation in many cancer patients that they barely developed a sense of their own identity as children. Fourth, that the spiritual connection has more often than not been based upon a certain set of rules and dogmas, lacking the freedom of an individual approach to faith, religion, or spirituality.

These are the kinds of amazing discoveries my clients and students make week after week, along with an increased awareness of how their individuality has been crushed by a system or society that expects a person to toe the line and act "normally".

Toeing the line and acting normally has led to the prediction that within one or two decades 50 percent of the Western world is expected to attract cancer. Some prospect to look forward to! Is that what you wish your future to be like? It's more or less a waiting game to see whether you are going to attract cancer or not. Waiting for the bad luck in the shape of a cancer diagnosis to arrive. Waiting to see on which side of the 50/50 dividing line you appear to be. To a large extent this dividing line is determined by you, your choices, your decisions, and your priorities.

In the words of Carl Gustav Jung, "To be normal is the ideal aim for the unsuccessful, for all those who are still below the general level of adaptation."

Success can be measured in terms of creative or social achievement, in wealth or in health.

Please realize, you are no different from the clients I have described. You are a human being who has had to make adjustments in order to live in society, to a larger or lesser degree—to what degree remains entirely your choice, and your choice alone. Ultimately, you are a physical human being with a human energy field and with human chakras. Your energetic self responds instantly to a change in thoughts, emotions, social surroundings, and environment to which your physical body reacts.

My wish is for this book to support you in awakening your awareness of who you really are, what you really wish for in life, and a way of exploring how your sense of identity has been underdeveloped and how that can be remedied. Self-awareness is essential in preventing illness, including cancer, for healing, and preventing illness from recurring.

References

Books

Bloom, William. *The Endorphin Effect: A Breakthrough Strategy for Holistic Health and Spiritual Well-being.* New York: Little Brown, 2011.

Brennan, Barbara. *Hands of Light: A Guide to Healing through the Human Energy Field.* New York: Bantam, 1988.

Collin-Smith, Joyce. *Call No Man Master.* South Lake, TX: Gateway, 2004.

Connor, Miriam. *Mary Had Stretch Marks: Honesty in Friendship is Feckin' Great.* Leicester, UK: Matador, 2013.

Dürckheim, Karlfried von. *Hara: The Vital Centre of Man.* New York: Mandala, 1977.

Eco, Umberto. *The Mysterious World of Queen Loana.* London: Vintage, 2006.

Edwards, Gill. *Conscious Medicine.* London: Piatkus, 2010.

Emoto, Masaru. *The True Power of Water: Healing and Discovering Ourselves.* New York: Atria Books, 2005.

Findhorn Community. *The Findhorn Garden: Pioneering a New Vision of Man and Nature in Cooperation.* Scotland: Findhorn Press, 1976. New edition: *The Findhorn Garden Story.* 2008.

Gerson, Dr. Max. *A Cancer Therapy: Results of 50 Cases and the Cure of Advanced Cancer by Diet Therapy.* 6th edition. San Diego, CA: The Gerson Institute, 2002.

Hay, Louise. *You Can Heal Your Life.* Carlsbad, CA: Hay House, 1985.

Jong, Tjitze de. *Cancer – A Healer's Perspective: Insights, Stories, and Messages of Hope.* Scott's Valley, CA: 2011.

Lowen, Alexander. *The Language of the Body.* New York: Macmillan, 1958.

Moerman, Dr. Cornelis. *A Solution to the Cancer Problem.* The Netherlands: The International Association of Cancer Victims and Friends, 1962.

Norwood, Robin. *Women Who Love Too Much: When You Keep Wishing and Hoping He'll Change.* NY: Pocket Books, 1985.

Pierrakos, John C. *Core Energetics: Developing the Capacity to Love and Heal.* Medocino, CA: Core Evolution Publishing, 2005.

Reich, Wilhelm. *Character Analysis.* Third Edition. New York: Farrar, Straus, and Giroux, 1980.

Rinpoche, Sogyal. *The Tibetan Book of Living and Dying.* San Francisco, CA: HarperSanFrancisco, 2020.

Schuitemaker, Lisette. *The Childhood Conclusions Fix: Turning Negative Self-Talk Around.* Scotland: Findhorn Press, 2017.

World Health Organization. *World Health Report 2003: Shaping the Future.* Geneva, Switzerland, World Health Organization, 2003.

Online Sources

Alexander, Ruth. "So, Is Cancer Mostly 'Bad Luck' or Not?" *BBC News Magazine.* (*https://www.bbc.com/news/magazine-30786970*)

Bollinger, Ty. *The Truth About Cancer: The Quest for the Cures Continues.* 11 episodes. *https://www.gaia.com/series/truth-about-cancer-quest -curescontinues.* Also available on PBS in the US.

Braden, Gregg. "Cancer Cured in Three Minutes." YouTube video. 29 April 2016. *https://www.youtube.com/watch?v=5suc-fz6PUk*

Burzynski, Stanislaw. *Burzynski, the Movie: Cancer Is Serious Business.* *https://vimeo.com/24821365*

Cancer Research UK. *www.cancerresearch.uk.gov*

Gerson, Max. Gerson Therapy. Hawaii Naturopathic Retreat. *www.hawaiinaturopathicretreat.com/procedures/gerson%20therapy*

Hamer, Ryke Geerd. The German New Medicine. *www.newmedicine.ca*

Moerman, Cornelis. *www.cancertutor.com/moerman*

Poponin, Vladimir. *www.researchgate.net*

Royal Rife, Raymond. *www.royal-rife-machine.com*

Tainio, Bruce. Tainio Biologicals, Inc. *www.tainio.com/about.*

Goldman Sachs. *Equity Research.* "Profiles in Innovation: The Genome Revolution." April 10, 2018. *https://www.gspublishing.com/content /research/en/reports/2019/09/04/048b0db6-996b-4b76-86f5 -0871641076fb.pdf*

Institute of Heart Math. *www.heartmath.org*

National Cancer Institute, US. *www.cancer.com*

"Sylvia Black: Life through Cancer". YouTube video. 17 January 2013. *https://www.youtube.com/watch?v=U8pylT3xhBk*

"Tjitze de Jong Sharing His Passion, videos 1–5". Glenn Moore's Passion Interviews. YouTube videos. 8–26 June 2016. *https://www.youtube.com /watch?v=IlJaUZ38Zck&t=26s*

Zabel, Barbie. blog "Science Says DNA Can Be Changed with
   FEELINGS: DNA Report by Gregg Braden." 7 November 2006.
   https://barbiezabel.blogspot.com/search?q=science+says+DNA

Schools for Energetic Cellular Healing

In 2007, I started the Bodies of Light certification programme in energetic cellular healing, later followed by Advanced BoL, where I also taught cancer healing work. After 12 years, I've decided to take a break from the intensity of teaching groups, and at present I am not sure whether I'll restart the school.

The following are the only schools where you can expect to study all of the healing techniques I offered in my own school:

Barbara Brennan School of Healing (*www.barbarabrennan.com*)
offers a four-year programme at schools situated in Miami, Florida, and Oxford, England. BBSH is in the process of opening branches in Istanbul, Turkey, and in Paris, France.

Centre for Integrative Development (*www.cir.hr*)
offers a four-year programme in Croatia.

Snowlion Center School (*www.snowlioncenterschool.com*)
offers a four-year programme in Italy.

Index